Bedtime Stories for Adults:

A Collection of Guided Relaxing Meditation Tales for Deep Sleep, Self-Healing, Self-Hypnosis, Letting Go of Stress, Anxiety & Insomnia to Fall Asleep Fast. For Grown-Ups

Daisy Relaxing

Please note the information contained within this document is for educational and entertainment purposes only.

All effort has been executed to present accurate, up to date, and reliable, complete information.

No warranties of any kind are declared or implied. Readers acknowledge that the author is not engaging in the rendering of legal, financial, medical or professional advice.

The content within this book has been derived from various sources. Please consult a licensed professional before attempting any techniques outlined in this book.

By reading this document, the reader agrees that under no circumstances is the author responsible for any losses, direct or indirect, which are incurred as a result of the use of the information contained within this document, including, but not limited to, — errors, omissions, or inaccuracies.

Table of Contents

Introduction

Congratulations on purchasing *Bedtime Stories for Adults: A Collection of Guided Relaxing Meditation Tales for Deep Sleep, Self-Healing & Self-Hypnosis. Letting Go of Stress, Anxiety, and Insomnia to Fall Asleep Fast. For Grown-Ups*

We all have moments of stress, deep concerns, anxiety, fear, and all kinds of thoughts and feelings that keep us awake at night.

These bedtime stories are a perfect resource for anyone who is looking for some solace and comfort, a way to shut off the churning thoughts of the mind to fully relax and let go of stress.

The following bedtime meditations will help you resolve the worries of the day and come to a final state of relaxation and peacefulness to help you drift off into a pleasant night's sleep.

Each meditation can be enjoyed on its own, or you can listen to several in a row on your way to deeper serenity.

The best way to enjoy this series of guided meditations is to find a soothing and comfortable place to relax in, turn off any distractions like television or cell phone alerts, and prepare to go into a deeper state of relaxation, healing, and rest.

All you have to do is lay back, relax, and listen as you get carried off into the depths of your unconscious to find release and relief through these creative visualizations and guided journeys into relaxation.

There are plenty of books on this subject on the market, thanks again for choosing this one! Every effort was made to ensure it is full of as much useful information as possible.

Please enjoy it!

Chapter 1: In the Garden of Wonders

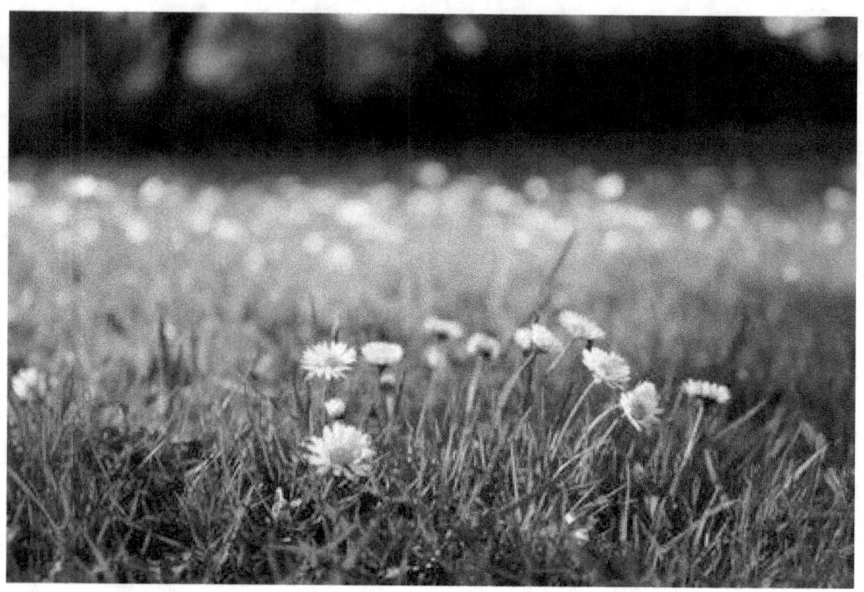

Collect your rest in the garden of wonders.

Find the enchantment of the hidden inner garden of your soul with this calming meditation and story for you to follow with your breath and your mind.

Find your comfort in relaxation as you walk in the landscape of abundance and peace.

Find a comfortable position and begin to connect to your breath.

Your breath is where you will always begin when you are ready to let go of your work, your worry, and your stress.

Your breath is where you begin to let go of the tension in your muscles, your joints, and your limbs.

Find your breath right now and let it flow naturally, in and out.

Inhale and exhale.

Bring your breath fully into your body on your next inhale, imagining the fresh oxygen circulating all the way down to your toes and all the way to the top of your head.

Feel yourself full of this cleansing breath until it is time to let it go, breathing out all of your tension and stress, letting your body melt into the surface you are laying on.

Allow a moment to let your body settle more deeply into the couch cushions or mattress.

Let each breath you draw into your lungs lift you out of your thoughts of concern or anxiety, breathing it all out and away from you as you settle more deeply into your comfort and relaxation.

Feel your body becoming heavier and heavier as you go deeper and deeper into relaxation, keeping your breath steady and smooth.

Allow all of the pain in your body, the strain, the muscle tension, to just melt away.

Exhale the discomforts you are feeling, the stressful conversation you had earlier today, the agenda, and the work.

Breathe it all out and resolve to enjoy only the soothing feeling of rest at this moment in time.

Connect to your inner mind and begin to see a small light.

With your eyes closed, see within your mind, picturing this small light getting brighter and bigger like you are walking toward a gateway or an open door.

All you can see is the growing light, a soft, warm, peachy glow that feels like a morning sunrise or an evening sunset.

Let yourself feel embraced by this warm, peachy light, growing bigger and bigger as you come closer to this place of light in your mind.

Let all of your cares peel off, like a snake shedding a skin, as you move closer to the growing light.

Continue to inhale and exhale slowly and deeply as you imagine this soft, warm glow.

Your inner mind is full of this light now, and as you get connected to your deeper relaxation, you can begin to see something in the distance of your mind.

A giant hedgerow that goes on and on in front of you, reaching up as tall as a tree, like a great long fence made of verdant, green leaves and branches, twirling all around each other and creating a barrier between you and the Garden of Wonders.

As you look upon this long thicket of twirling, intersecting branches and leaves, you spot a colorful object.

From where you stand, it just looks like something buried in the branches.

You start to walk closer to see what it is, the warm peach glow of light still embracing you in this landscape.

As you get closer and closer to this colorful object hidden in the branches, you push some of the foliage away to get a better glimpse of what it is peaking out at you.

You see that it has a doorknob attached to it.

The doorknob is ornate and looks very old and intricate.

This hedgerow has a hidden doorway inside of it, leading you to another place, and all you have to do is turn the doorknob and push the door open to discover what is beyond the wall of winding branches.

You turn the knob, and it creaks and groans to life.

You hear a click and feel the readiness for the door to be pushed open.

You can feel yourself getting excited to explore what is on the other side.

The door swings open, and you must duck down to walk under the overgrown branches surrounding it to get through to the other side.

You push your way through, closing the door behind you.

As you begin to look around the world you have entered, your eyes are full to the brim with the most magical colors, sounds, plants and flowers, creatures, and natural world elements.

It is like no garden you have seen before.

It is the garden of your mind, of your memories, of your imagination.

It is your unique inner garden that shows you more of who you are and what you need from deep within.

You are alone in this space and are free to just breathe and relax.

There is no work to do here.

There is no agenda.

The only thing that you have to do here is rest and relax.

Underneath your feet, as you look down to the ground, the earth is covered in soft, green, velvety moss.

Your feet can feel this softness, like a comfortable blanket laid out before you to enjoy as you walk.

You can hear the soft rustle of the moss under your feet as you approach a pond surrounded by exotic flowers.

Your body floats effortlessly down to a seated position, leaning against a soft patch of mossy ground.

There beside you, deep in the black waters of the rippling pond, you see fat, round coy fish, slowly flicking their tales and swimming through the water.

They are brightly colored and easy to spot in the murky water.

You notice the lily pads floating on top of the pond and how they wobble gently with every ripple of the water's surface.

A cluster of dragonflies is hovering around the pond.

One of them lands on a lily pad on the pond water.

Its wings and body are emerald and iridescent, gathering the light of the peachy warm glow and reflecting it.

You spend a moment enjoying the hum of the dragonflies floating around, and the swirl of the coy fish in the pond, taking in the calmness of the surrounding garden.

From here, looking around this enclosed garden of wonders, you see a multi-colored carpet of various flowers, shrubs, and trees.

Every color looks more saturated than anything you have ever seen.

Each flower almost looks like it is made of confection, soft and fluffy, and almost good enough to eat.

You stand up from the pond and begin to wander gently through the flowers.

There are thousands of them all around you now as you walk closer to where they are all growing together.

It is almost as if you are swimming in an ocean of colorful flowers, all of which are soft and delicate and inviting you to touch them.

Each flower has such sweet softness.

As you reach out a hand to caress a flower, it moves closer to you and rubs against your skin, caressing you first.

The flowers all around you begin to hold you, coming closer and swirling around you, like a cyclone of colorful love.

It is slow and gentle, like a river flowing softly around your skin.

All of a sudden, you feel the current of soft and colorful flowers swirling gently around you, lifting your feet off of the ground and carrying you up and away.

The encircling flowers feel like ten thousand butterflies flitting around you like a school of fish, transporting you to somewhere new in the garden.

You float through this swirl of soft comfort until you begin to feel yourself begin carefully lowered to somewhere else on the ground, somewhere deeply soft and relaxing, somewhere that you feel secure and safe and composed.

As the swirl of flowers that carried you here covers the land around you, you begin to notice a starlit sky above you.

It is now night, and your journey into the garden has carried you to this special, quiet landscape hidden under the stars.

The ground underneath you where you are laying down in soft moss and rose petals.

The air around you is just the right temperature to help you feel warm and safe.

Looking around the garden, you notice the quiet calm of all of the plants and flowers in their silver moonlight resting state.

They are peaceful and grounded, deeply rooted in the earth.

They are bathing in starlight, and as you welcome the energy of their serenity, you become like the flowers and plants that surround you: calm, quiet, peaceful, gentle, serene.

You can feel the whimsy and enchantment of this inner garden, this majestic world, untouched by civilization.

It is alive and free within the borders of the twisting branches and vines that enclose it.

As you lay comfortably here, you sense the presence of a vine beginning to curl around your ankle, like a gentle hand, holding you and letting you know that you are held by the garden.

You are safe here.

You feel the vines wrap softly around you like a warm blanket or a comforting hug from a friend.

Take a deep breath and relax into this energy.

The energy of being held by the forest and the trees, the stars, the plants, the animals.

Exhale slowly and let yourself sink even more deeply into your relaxed state of inner peace and calm.

Your heart feels open and full of light in this place.

You feel content and at ease.

There are no worries to contend with.

You are free to relax here.

You are safe and held by this mysterious garden.

The forest creatures, which have soft eyes and gentle qualities, emerge from their burrows to quietly gather around you and hold space for you here.

They welcome you with their heartbeats, with the flap of their soft wings.

They all become relaxed with you, curling up for a peaceful and pleasant rest in the Garden of Wonders.

As you lay in this position, under the stars, wrapped in the comfort of growing vines, surrounded by gentle creatures, you begin to feel the warm, peach glow filling your heart.

The light is coming from inside of you and expanding as you take a deep breath in and let it grow bigger and bigger inside of you.

The peach light is your peacefulness, your serenity, your calm.

It has entered you in this space of rejuvenation and release.

As you fell the warmth of this light, see it starting in your heart and then radiating from there through your whole being.

Fill your body with peach light and let yourself bathe in the comfort of this energy.

See it pumping through your veins like blood, circulating into every system, every organ, every cell.

Take a deep breath in, allowing your peach glow to ground you to the mossy, rose-covered ground you are laying on.

As you exhale, breathe the peach light out into your garden of wonders.

See this soothing, warm light beginning to spread like a blanket of soothing comfort.

Inhale in, grounding your body to the soft moss beneath you, exhaling soothing peach light into the garden around you.

Let it fill the flowers, the plants, the trees.

See it embracing and enveloping the peaceful animals that surround you and keep you safe.

Inhale, pulling the magic of the starlight into your heart.

Exhale the warm light into the garden until the whole space is filled: the pond, the fish, the water, the flowers, the branches and twigs, the skyline...

Continue to inhale and exhale peach-colored warmth into your garden of wonders for a few moments...

Your light has filled the space around you in this magical garden.

You are safe and held here. You are protected and free to just sleep and relax.

You have nothing you need to think about now, nothing to fear or worry.

There is nothing that you have to accomplish, nothing that needs attention.

It is all resting.

It is all asleep.

The garden of wonders is quiet and calm, resting with you.

The essence of time has drifted away.

You do not need a clock to rest in this garden.

You do not need anything to tell you when to stop resting and relaxing.

You are safe to just sleep in this space, wrapped up in soothing, friendly vines, comforted by the creatures nearby, held by your own inner light and warmth.

Your world is full of this power.

It is time to rest your eyes, your mind, your thoughts.

It is time to let go of your cares and concerns.

It is time to let go of time and just rest.

Feel your body go deeper into this space.

You are not going to get up for a while.

You are going to lay here and enjoy the serenity of this garden and all that it can give to you.

You are just going to sleep, breathe, dream.

You are ready to find your dreamland.

You are ready to let go of the outside world and explore your inner mind through your dreams.

Release yourself and let go.

Go further into your garden of wonders now.

Take your time.

Move slowly through your peachy warmth.

Breathe and let your unconscious mind transport you even deeper into this state of calm and peacefulness.

Take a long time to connect to your breath, to your comfort, to your softened mind and body.

Let yourself feel heavy and sunken into the soft, warm moss and earth.

Let yourself feel fully held by the vines blanketing you.

Let yourself release into comfort and rest.

It is time now to just drift off...go deeper...and deeper....and deeper.

Fall further and further...all the way into peaceful sleep...

Chapter 2: The Hidden Cave

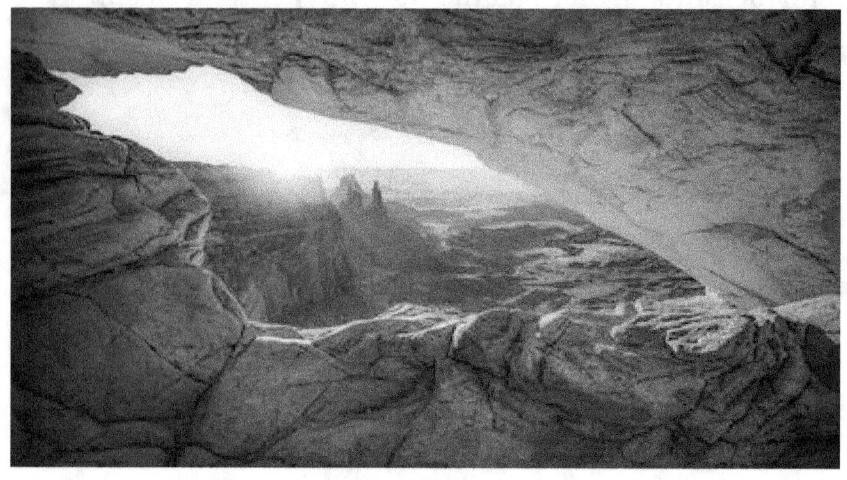

A cave is always such a mysterious place.

A cave is where you will find buried treasures and unlikely beauty.

A cave can also be the place deep inside of you where you hide all of your deepest desires and darkest fears.

In your next bedtime story and guided meditation, you will travel to a hidden cave of mystery to find just what your mind, heart, and soul need in order for you to feel free, relaxed, and relieved.

Begin by finding your most comfortable position.

If you are preparing for bed and ready for this bedtime story, make sure you have everything you will need to feel settled.

As you get comfortable in your space, connect to your breath and begin to listen to the flow of air being pulled in through your nostrils, being held in your chest for a moment's pause, and releasing your breath in one, long exhale.

Breathe in again, pulling in clarity, calmness, serenity, hold it here in your lungs, and exhale it out.

Breathe like this for a few moments and make any final adjustments you need to in order to find the most comfortable position for your body.

As you breathe in and out, connect to your sense and feeling.

How is your body feeling right now?

Where do you feel stiffness, soreness, achiness?

Where do you feel tightness, or like you are holding onto something that needs to be released?

When you find these spaces in your body, breathe into them with your inhale, filling the space with clean, clear oxygen.

Hold the breath in this area for a moment, and release it slowly and steadily out.

Again, find these spaces of tension, of soreness, or tightness.

Breathe long, slow, soothing breaths into these areas, hold the breath here for a moment and then let it all out in a long, steady exhale.

Feel your body becoming heavier and more relaxed as you breathe out your tension.

Feel your body sinking more deeply into the relaxed position you are laying in right now.

Feel your body acclimate to this restful state.

Notice how it feels when it is free of tension.

Notice how it feels after focused breathing.

Your body and mind are linked.

It is one.

Everything that you think, your body can hear it, feel it, sense it.

All of your emotions, your fears, your anxieties, all of your trauma, sadness, frustration, all of these things become a part of your physical self.

All of these mental patterns and beliefs become a part of your physical form, the way you carry yourself, the way your shoulders and neck tighten.

Continue to breathe in and out and feel your body melt and become relaxed, like honey dripping from a honeycomb.

See your muscles and ligaments, joints, and bones, becoming thick and fluid, like golden honey.

Feel your body relaxing in this way with every release of tension or tightness as you exhale slowly.

Now, once upon a time, you saw a starry night.

It was the first thing you saw when you opened your inner eye.

In your mind, see the starry night sky.

You are there now.

You are laying underneath a great, wide expanse of stars.

The sky is rich and full of these burning bulbs, millions of miles away.

You are in a place where you can see all of the stars of the night sky.

It is the only light.

Your body is calm and liquid, and your mind is seeing this space, this expanse of stars.

Your energy can feel the power of this starlight beaming down and touching the landscape that surrounds you, wherever you are laying.

This starry sky reaches across and over everything, as far as your eye can see, from horizon to horizon.

There is no end to it.

What kind of landscape do you find yourself in?

A desert canyon?

A pine forest?

A meadow?

A prairie?

Where did your mind transport you to view this starry night sky?

Look around inside your mind at this space.

What is beneath the sky of stars, other than your body?

It can be anything and everything you can imagine...

This place you are in, it is real.

It exists inside of you.

It is a place that your mind can see and that you can travel to with your consciousness.

You can see it change and evolve as you change and evolve, and it will always contain everything you need to explore your deeper mind.

This is your conscious reality in your unconscious mind space.

Take it in and let it be whatever comes to your mind.

This space you are in has always existed and always will.

It is a place of good intentions and dreams.

It is a place of fearlessness and awakening.

It is a place you will go to whenever you need to find what you are looking for to help you forward on your healing path.

Let it begin to take new shape in your mind as it changes from starry night to dawn's light.

See the sun rising on a horizon, bringing new energy to this landscape.

As the sun begins to rise, you can begin to walk toward the pink and orange light of sunrise.

Let your body float across the landscape, continuing to feel fluid like honey.

Feel yourself being naturally guided and carried forward in this landscape of your inner mind and thoughts.

Let the world around you take new shape as you gently explore its features.

You are walking to a distant space near the horizon.

You see far off in the distance a flickering light.

You are drawn to it like a bee to pollen, or a moth to a flame.

You walk toward it.

As you get closer and closer, the dawn turns into day, and the day turns to dusk, and the dusk turns to night again, blanketing the night sky with stars as far as the eye can see.

The flickering light is now close to you.

As you draw nearer under the stars, you see that it is a campfire that someone built and left all alone.

As you come closer to it, you feel its warmth and the orange glow on your cheeks.

It feels good to be here under the stars in this land next to the warm, passionate glow of the fire.

You can hear the crack and hiss of the burning embers, and you feel this fire awakening within you, warming you from your very core, aligning with your own burning flame.

This fire you found under the stars is a reflection of your internal flame.

How does your internal flame feel today?

Is it burning brightly?

Does it lack fuel?

Do you feel it growing as you relax in this inner landscape?

Take a deep breath in and allow the power of flame to fill your soul, warming the liquid honey of your body.

Exhale slowly and look out into the distance, all-around your inner world, feeling the calm of everything you have created in your subconscious wilderness.

Underneath this starry night, the world is full of hidden mysteries and secrets to be unearthed.

Your greatest desires and needs are here in this place.

Can you look for them here? Can you sense which direction you need to walk in order to find your hidden cave of answers?

Let yourself feel pulled forward in a direction.

Walk away from the glow of the firelight and let yourself journey toward this hidden place that is waiting for you to come.

Continue your journey, breathing softly and deeply, letting the radiance of each star glimmer on your skin from far off in the galaxy.

Let your honey-body glide and float without any tension or fear.

See the place where you know the cave might be hidden and follow your path there.

Your path to this cave can be anything you want.

As you draw nearer to where you feel pulled, you find yourself in a canyon with high rock walls.

Let your mind fill in this space with color, with detail, with scope.

This rocky canyon holds many deep mysteries and energies from deep within your mind.

As you walk through this canyon, you are still being pulled toward this source of power, somewhere hidden, deep in the caves of your consciousness.

It's somewhere here, the opening.

It blends in so well to the rock walls because you are so good at keeping it safe and hidden from others.

You are looking for the opening of the cave when you spot a small stone on the surface where you are gliding.

The stone is a beautiful color and is perfectly smooth.

It fits in your palm and feels like a comfortable and soothing weight.

Its cool exterior warms in the palm of your hand.

You notice its color and its shape as you hold it, and somehow you know that this stone is the key to finding the hidden cave.

This stone marks the entrance somewhere close by.

In your eye, you can see the possibilities of where this hidden entrance might be.

You can glance around now and try to spot it.

Look for a sign that will show you the path to the hidden entrance.

Is it another colorful stone marking the gateway?

Is it perhaps a secret message carved in the rock wall?

Seek the sign to show you the door to the cave.

Welcome the energy of the cave by finding the entrance.

The entrance will become obvious once you see it, and once you see it, it opens wide for you, like the mouth of a yawning lion.

You can see the tunnel that opens into the deep of this canyon wall.

You are free to walk toward it and enter the mysteries that are hidden here.

Are you ready to walk the path?

There is nothing to fear as you enter the tunnel of the cave.

It is open and welcoming to you.

It is a part of your thoughts, your soul, your mind.

It feels right.

It feels natural.

It is a place within you that is hiding something of great value to you on your journey of healing and self-discovery.

Let yourself flow into the tunnel opening of the cave and follow the path.

You can see where you are going because the walls of the cave are glittering and alive with bioluminescence.

Blue-green light, purple light, white light, shimmers from the life forms that grow in this magic place.

You are being shown the way down your path by this organic light source, and you are brave enough to keep walking straight through the winding and crooked pathways carved into the walls of the cave.

There is nowhere inside where you will be stuck or won't be able to get out.

This cave is a friend to you and your sense of self.

It is a part of you, this cave.

It is a reflection of your subconscious thoughts and feelings.

Let it become what it wants to be so that you can see your true mind inside of the shadows of this cave.

You are nearing an opening, a large chamber at the center of the cave maze.

You can feel the air opening up here.

You can hear the echo of dripping water hitting the floor of the cave as it falls from stalactites growing off the ceiling, hanging down like chandeliers of water and light.

There are crystals growing in all directions in this chamber, adding to the light of the space.

They are white, clear, purple, and other colors of quartz growing out of walls, the cave floor, the ceiling.

You are surrounded by the vibration of these crystals.

You can feel them humming in soft tones, filling the space with the frequency of love.

You are safe and guarded by the energy of this space.

As you walk into the center of the cave, surrounded by all of the crystals, you see a large wooden chest with a lock on it.

The lock is in the shape of the colorful stone you found outside the cave opening.

You can open this wooden chest with the colorful rock that showed you where to find the hidden cave.

You approach the wooden chest and kneel on the floor in front of it.

Notice its features.

How big is it?

How worn and used?

What does it fell like when you touch it?

Take a deep breath in and consider what this chest feels like to you on the outside, exhaling as you reflect on it.

Inhale again and consider what might be locked inside.

What is within this chest hidden in your cave of mysterious?

What have you come to find?

What are you looking for that you didn't even realize was hidden?

Take a moment to reflect in this space, surrounded by crystals and bioluminescence.

Breathe gently and slowly, in and out.

Consider what you need to open in your life, something buried deep within that needs to come to the surface that needs to be awakened in your everyday existence.

You have a colorful stone with you.

It is in the palm of your hand.

You can open the lock of the chest with the stone.

The stone slides snugly into an opening in this strange lock.

You hear it click open and fall from the chest onto the cave floor.

The chest is now unlocked, and you can look inside to find what you need right now.

All you have to do is lift the lid and look inside.

Let it come to you naturally.

Do not guess.

Let the hidden item, or emotion, or memory, or experience, organically take shape as you open the chest and look inside.

If it takes a moment to materialize, that's okay.

It might be a small object.

It could be an entire person, you know.

It might look like a symbol of what you want or desire.

Only you will know.

Only you can see it.

Take a few moments to look inside the chest and find the hidden gift.

Whatever it is, it is now time for you to look at it in the cave.

If you find something you were not expecting, you are on the right track.

If you found something you were expecting to find, then you are also on the right track.

The hidden cave of mysterious shows you what you need to see right now, today, to help you align with your higher purpose, your wholeness, your growth.

Whatever you have found in this treasure chest is what will help you heal and find peacefulness from within.

It could be a lost passion or a hidden desire.

It could be a relationship that needs to end or begin anew.

It could be a profession that has been calling to you for years or a career that is at a dead end.

It could be an old object from childhood that is the key to rekindling your childlike curiosity.

It could be a memory that hides your greatest pain or your deepest love.

It is time to acknowledge your feelings about this hidden truth.

It is time to accept what it is you are hiding or blocking from being seen or heard, or recognized.

This hidden artifact of your subconscious mind is asking to be held by you, is asking to be given more attention.

Whatever emotions are connected to it, any beliefs or attitudes that might come up with it, are important to see also.

Let yourself spend time examining this hidden energy that you have kept locked in this hidden cave deep within your mind.

This energy that you have held onto is ready to be shown out of the cave, to be bathed in the starlight and the rising dawn.

You can shrink it down and hold it in your hand, carrying the essence of it out of the cave with you.

You can close the lid of the trunk and lock it again.

You will return to it again sometime soon, and it will contain another hidden treasure for you to open.

Let your breath relax you as you begin your ascent out of the cave, touching the giant crystals to give you balance along the way, soaking in the subtle glow of the bioluminescent organisms clinging to the cave walls, lighting your way out.

The cave is narrowing behind you as you exit, hiding again until it is time for your return.

The opening of the cave closes as you take your final step back out into the canyon, like the jaws of the yawning lion closing again.

You are back underneath the starlight, and you are holding the essence of your hidden mystery in your hand. In your other hand, the colorful stone is warm and weighted.

You drop it on the ground and leave it there for your next visit, carrying only the essence of your hidden mystery in your hand.

It is time to let it see the light of day, out of the cave walls, out of the buried and locked chest.

Hold this energy in your hand and carry it with you through the canyon, following the starlight as it changes into a morning sunrise.

You can see the flickering campfire still flickering with life on the distant horizon.

Walk to it, breathing in gently and softly, relaxing your body, keeping it like honey flowing smoothly.

As you near the fire, you approach it with good intentions.

This hidden secret you have locked inside of you is ready to be transformed.

It is time to give it to the light and let it evolve and grow in the way it asks to, as you welcome it into your higher consciousness.

Whatever you have pulled from the secret chest in the hidden cave, whether it is positive or negative, is asking to be turned over to the fire of the dawn.

Lifting your hand high, hold the essence of your hidden secret above the flames.

Hold it up to the disappearing starlight and the waking sun.

Show this energy that you found locked deep inside of you that you are ready to set it afire so that it can change so that it can grow so that it can go through metamorphosis.

You are ready to let your inner light shine brighter by giving this locked secret to the fire.

Take a deep breath in, slowly inhaling, filling yourself with empowered energy.

As you exhale, see yourself dropping the image or essence of your hidden mystery into the flames.

Hear it crackle and hiss.

Hear it burn and transform.

This is where you start fresh.

This is where you can begin anew.

You are ready to seek out new ideas, new energy, new comfort, just by letting go of this secret energy to the flame of creation, passion, and desire.

You are burning an opening into your journey so that you can have new momentum, new life-force, new excitement.

You can now relax as the sun comes forward and warms you like the flame you sit beside.

Lay down next to the fire.

Feel the starlight on your back and the dawn's light on your face.

Breathe in slowly and smoothly and give yourself the peace to relax and dream of what tomorrow will bring.

Feel the relief of knowing where to find your hidden cave anytime you need to resolve a buried intention.

Let yourself burrow into the earth where you are laying in front of the fire.

Relax.

Dream.

Rest.

Sleep.....

Chapter 3: The Secret Map

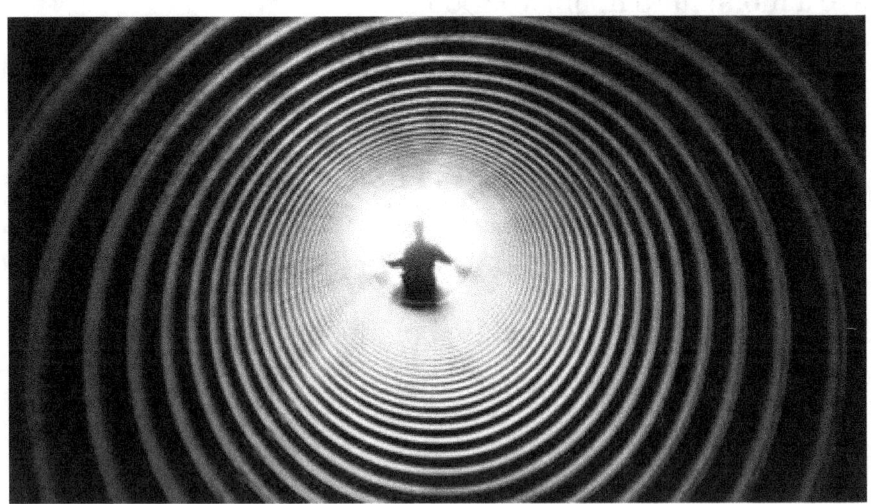

You are alone in your bed or your space of comfort.

You are here to rest and relax.

There is nothing left to do now but just sink into the covers, melt into the mattress, and find relief in your body after a long day.

You are here to fully inspire total serenity, peace of mind, and relaxation.

Anything you need to do to find your most comfortable resting position do so now...

Take a moment to honor your body.

Find your stillness and your center.

Let go of any judgments you have about your body or the way it feels.

Simply notice the areas that are holding onto something or that have tension, and let it all flow out when you exhale.

Your body can begin to rest.

Underneath all of the layers of your day, your work, your relationships, your tasks or deadlines, there is just quiet space.

In this bedtime story, you are going to find a secret map that will take you to this place of quiet and release so that you can find a deeper comfort from within you.

You hold the key to your relief, and this guided meditation and bedtime visualization will take you there, one step at a time.

Your breath should start to become long... slow...and steady.

Let it flow naturally.

Don't overthink your breathing.

Just allow it to transport you more deeply into your relaxed state of mind and body.

Your physical self has been at work all day.

Even if you weren't moving around all that much, if you had to sit down at your desk, or work from a seated position somewhere, your whole body has still worked hard.

Your mind has been hard at work, even when you are at play.

You are always thinking, weighing and calculating, observing, listening, processing.

You have all of the energy of thought radiating from your brain and from your body.

Now, you can begin to let your energy flow in longer, thicker waves.

You no longer need to be at attention.

You are now available to sink into a state of total relaxation.

Help your body feel softer and more elastic with each inhale of breath, and each exhale of tension or any kind of thoughts or ideas that keep circling around.

Breathe it all out and come to a place of peace of mind...and body.

You are now in a more relaxed state of energy, and you can fall even deeper into your unconsciousness.

You are ready to take a journey farther than you have ever traveled before.

You are ready to discover your highest state of relief, your most sacred level of self-healing, finding your balance with every breath as you transcend space, time, and the material world.

Begin to see in your mind a bright light at the end of a long tunnel.

The tunnel is a part of your mind that takes you into a deeper layer of your consciousness.

You can float through the tunnel, like a seed in the wind, going closer to the light at the end, feeling yourself soften, and welcome the spiral of light that opens before you...

The tunnel is widening as you come fully into the light.

Feel it surround you, almost blinding you from what lies on the other side.

The light is so bright that it fills your whole being, penetrating your skin, and filling you with healing warmth and love.

You can feel it with every breath you inhale, the light filling your lungs, and circulating through your body.

As you exhale now, you will feel the brightness of the light normalize, opening your sight to see a great open meadow covered in soft green grass and flowers dancing on a soft breeze.

The air around you is crisp and clear, clean, and cool, but your body remains warm, safe, protected.

You can see a wide range of snow-capped mountains surrounding the meadow.

It is bright and open, full of possibilities.

You are here in this space, a place of your deeper mind.

You are free to explore this land, this mountain range, this secret world.

You feel an urge to explore in several directions, and you aren't quite sure where to begin.

There are many potential paths to explore, many ways you can go to find your deepest calm and relaxation.

If only you had a map, a map that could point you in the right direction, a map that would hold you close and give you everything you need to explore this place and guide you to your serenity.

As you ponder this, you feel a tingle in your palms.

Lifting up your hands, you notice that there are markings where there were none before.

The markings are starting to make sense.

A map is imprinted on your palms.

It shows you exactly where you need to go.

Your healing path is always in your hands, and all you have to do is trust yourself that you already know where you need to go in order to find inner harmony and peace.

The map on your hands is showing you a path to walk.

You look up at the mountains and the meadow, and you find the direction your hands are pointing you toward.

Follow the arrows of your inner mind.

Follow the way you are showing yourself to travel.

Walk in that direction, noticing the place you are and how it feels to have awareness in your deeper mind.

Inhale deeply and let out a long, slow breath.

Let your body remain relaxed, peaceful, serene, as your mind travels to these inner pathways.

Perhaps a fog thickens on your path, or maybe there is a soothing river flowing across your path.

Let the natural world of your mind unfold.

If you are uncertain of where to travel, look down at the map on your hands for guidance.

Trust your intuition to show you the path...

As you continue to breathe and follow your secret map forward, let yourself begin to seek even further down into your subconscious mind.

The landscape, the dreamscape, the world of your mind can become anything you want it to be.

Where is it leading you?

What is happening on your path as you follow the secret map of your soul and your mind?

Is it still comforting and pleasant?

Do you feel like your map has taken you on a darker road, a more shadowy path? A

re you still following the map of yourself to find where to go?

If you begin to feel like you are getting off the path, or if you feel like you are leading yourself into dark territory, that's okay.

Sometimes that can be exactly where you need to travel in order to heal your deeper self and your deeper mind.

If you need to get back on a lighter path, you can take a few soothing breaths in and out, and let the sun come out and beam bright, warm, healing light onto the shadows of your mind.

Let the map continue to show you the way you need to go.

Underneath the power of your journey lies the answer to where your inner harmony lives and breathes.

Somewhere the map of your consciousness is the answer to how to heal yourself on the deepest level.

Your secret map is always working with you to help you find your path.

Now, look down at the map on your hands.

Look to see if there is an 'X' that marks the end of your quest in this sacred wilderness deep within your mind.

Do you see it?

How are you going to get there?

How will the path take you to the 'X' on the map?

Looking around, can you see where you want to go?

Can you sense where that X is inside of this place?

Go there.

Seek it out.

Find the X from the palm of your hand in the land of your mind, in the place of your soul and your subconscious.

Perhaps it is a very direct path.

Perhaps it is winding and bending.

Maybe you need to climb over a few obstacles here and there, or perhaps you encounter a challenge along the road.

Keep going.

When in doubt, look at the map on your hand.

Let it lead you to the X that marks the spot… (take several moments to search for it).

You are now around the spot where your final destination is laid.

You have found the ground where the 'X' is painted or etched on the earth or on a tree.

Perhaps it is carved in the rocks of the mountainside, or it could be less obvious and more like a feeling that you just know that this is the place.

What does this place look like?

How does it feel to be here?

How long did it take you to find it?

Inhale deeply, taking a long soothing breath of air into your body.

Hold it for a moment, and now exhale slowly, steadily letting the air leave you.

And inhale again, filling yourself with the feeling of discovery, the feeling of finding the spot on your map.

Exhale slowly, going deeper into your mind, deeper into your fullness and relaxed state.

Here is where your healing can begin, when you let go of all of the other spaces outside of you, when you seek out your 'X' on your inner map, as it guides you into the deepest points of growth and transformation, the deepest points of total relaxation and relief.

Here is where you can release judgment and critique.

Here is where you can enlist your power to resolve the hardest moments and the biggest challenges.

Let your body sink into this space.

Let your heart open to finding resolve so that you can feel at peace.

Your mind is made of thoughts and beliefs, attitudes, and emotions.

Your mind is also made of spirit, your spirit—the life force energy that gives you the secret map of your inner journey.

Your spirit aligns you with your purpose and the right path for you, directing you along the way, a new direction every day.

All you have to do is find your focus and follow the map to where your 'X' marks the spot.

This map has led you to a place of total peace and inner harmony.

You are here to rest, sleep, dream.

You are here to fall deeply into serenity and balance.

In the space, deep within your subconscious mind, you now see a door.

This door is familiar to you, and you know that it will lead you back home, back to the security of your warm bed, back to your whole body and mind.

When you walk through this door, all you have to do is rest.

All you have to do is sleep. All you have to do is dream of where your secret map will lead you next.

Walkthrough the door...sink deeply into your mattress or cushions...go deeply into the dreamworld...until the next map leads you to where you need to be...

Chapter 4: The Place of Greatest Comfort

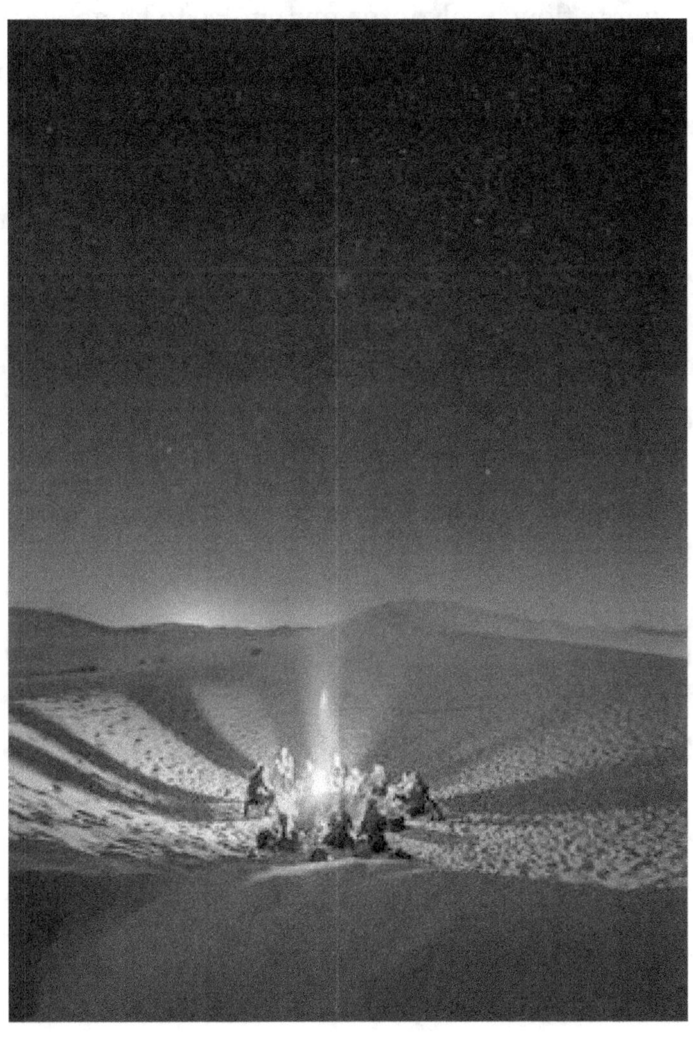

Welcome your breath as you find your relaxed state of mind and body.

Let your energy flow freely into your choice to let go, lay down, take comfort, and find solitude in the night hours, or before a long rest.

Prepare your body, your thoughts, your emotions, to fall forward into relief and inner comfort.

Let your soul feel prepared to feel held warmly by loving energy and inner light.

Take a few deep breaths in and exhale out to align with your comfort.

Help your body feel snuggled in and at peace.

Find all of the soft cushions and blankets you need to feel at home and at peace.

You are going to become more and more relaxed with every breath you take.

With every inhale, refresh your body with new oxygen, new energy, cleansing, and purifying your inner world. With every exhale, release all of the tension from your body and your thoughts.

Release your worries and concerns.

Breathe in comfort, peace of mind, serenity.

Breathe out stress and worry, negativity, and pain.

As you connect further to your relaxed state of mind, feel soothed and nurtured by your choice to take time for a bedtime story.

Acknowledge that you are taking good care of yourself right now, at this moment.

Acknowledge that you are nurturing yourself back to health and giving yourself space to heal and rejuvenate.

Going deeper into this restful state, connect to your warmest memories of home, your most filling spaces you've known.

Connect to your places of greatest comfort in your mind and start to see in your third eye what that space looks like.

Open your heart and your mind to the part of your wholeness that feels the safest, the most comfortable, the most nurtured.

It could be your childhood home, or perhaps the space you live in now.

Maybe it is a beloved holiday memory or a film that gives you comfort.

It may be as simple as a picture in your mind of an old country cottage with a crackling fire and a pot of stew simmering on the stove.

Let your mind form this place of greatest comfort.

Take a few moments, breathing in slowly, letting it out steadily, and picture this serene and wholesome place...

You are here to find solace and inner harmony.

This dwelling space you are in that feels comforting to you is where you have come to feel at ease.

This is where you can become well again, nurtured, warmed by the fire.

This is where you will be fed by loved ones, family friends, or even your spiritual guides who have come to hold space for you.

When you take a look around this space, who is here to give you comfort?

What energies have come to support you and keep you safe and warm?

It can be anyone.

It can be anything.

Let your subconscious mind welcome whatever comes to give you balance and inner peace...

Continue to lay in this space, snuggled into your warm blankets, cozy and comforted as you welcome these energies, whether they are people or spirits.

What does it feel like to be surrounded by a warm, loving company?

How does it feel to have a place to just lay down and be taken care of?

You have no obligations here, no one to take care of.

You are the one being cared for.

You are the one who is being nurtured and loved.

Let the spirits and people who have traveled to this place in your heart gather around you and give you love and attention.

Feel their soft, friendly smiles giving you comfort and openness in your soul and mind.

As you continue to rest in the space of great comfort, the people, friends, allies, spirit guides, or others who have come to nurture and care for you are beginning to prepare a feast of the most nutritious and nourishing food.

All of your favorite foods that will heal you and make you feel whole.

You can hear the sound of foods being chopped, the sound of boiling soup on the stove, the aroma of fresh ingredients.

They are here to help you feel well taken care of, loved.

They are roasting things in the oven, the smell filling the whole space.

They are stirring the logs on the fire and making sure your blankets are tucked in.

Keeping you warm and cozy.

You have everything you need here.

You can just be.

You are being taken care of and loved in this place of greatest comfort.

The feeling that surrounds you is that of being held by all of the things that make you feel warm, whole, heart-felt, and secure.

The foods being prepared are the ones that make you feel nurtured and nourished.

The pleasantness of this place is what feels so healing and good.

It is your inner home and that good feeling that comes from your wholeness within.

As you are laying there, swaddled in blankets, taking in the aroma of your favorite dishes being prepared and the sounds of laughter and loving energy coming from those who have gathered, you feel someone lift you up and carry you, wrapped in warmth, to a table where there are many places laid for you and all of your company to share a delicious meal by a warm, glowing fire.

As you look from one end of the table to the other, it feels endless.

The candles are lit.

There is food on every inch of the table: fresh-baked bread, still hot from the oven, bowls of fresh fruits and herbs, homemade cookies, goblets of delicious drinks, roasted dishes, everything your heart desires, laid out in front of you.

You are surrounded by the love and affection of whoever is here with you.

The fire is crackling, and someone adds another log to keep it going.

As you look around the table at the feast, at your family and friends, your spiritual guides, you are filled with a sense of warmth and wonder.

There is nothing but kindness and generosity here, and you have no other concerns.

Everyone is merry and filling up on the wonderfully nutritious and nourishing foods.

You feel at peace, connected to this moment, to these friends and allies, to this meal.

When you are finished eating, and you glance around the table, you can sense and feel the contentedness of those around you, and it fills your heart with joy and tenderness.

You are warm in your blankets, full of the glorious feast, and held by the family that surrounds you.

You are free to just relax and breathe for a few moments, taking in this feeling of true peace and serenity.

Just as you feel like you could drift off to sleep, you feel someone lift you up again and carry you over to a soft, cushioned sofa near the fire.

You are tucked gently into your blankets, swaddled like a baby as the others gather around the sitting place near the fire.

Everyone is together for a delightful story to help everyone drift off into a safe and comfortable world of dreams.

You listen to the story as it begins.

Nothing feels more pleasant than having this comfort, this warmth, this generosity of spirit.

You can sense the blissfulness of everyone gathering together for a story to continue relaxing and feeling connected to the place of greatest comfort.

Your breath is slow and steady and deep.

You have nothing to think about or control in this place.

You have nothing to worry about, no problems to solve.

You are totally free to just relax and exist in the warmth of this space with these loving energies holding and embracing you.

As the story begins to unfold, you feel a release from deep within that lets you know that you are free to fall asleep anytime you feel like it.

You are welcome to listen until your body and mind float away, deeper and deeper into the world of dreams, into total relaxation and healing.

The story begins to take shape in your ears as you snuggle tightly into your covers, surrounded by the warm, healing light of the fire and the sense that you are not alone, that you are protected by those that surround you.

It begins as you take a deep breath in and sigh it out with relief...

Once upon a time, there was a cottage nestled deep in a forest.

The forest was very old, and the trees had been listening to all of the life within the forest for thousands of years.

The cottage had been there for a long time too, and tonight it was full of love and warmth and serenity.

The people inside of the cottage were baking loaves of bread and sweets, stirring a large pot of stew, and feasting on the delicious flavors of Autumn time as the nights grew colder and the wind blew harder, whispering of the winter to come.

The feast was fragrant and sumptuous.

The taste of every bite was fulfilling.

Every nibble of soft, warm bread felt soothing to the soul; every sip of hot broth was warming to the heart.

The candles burned, and the warm glow of firelight permeated to simple cottage walls, giving peace and comfort to all who sat at the table.

All around there was laughter and kindness and friendship.

All around there was life and beauty and harmony.

The people sitting at the table felt satiated and at peace.

It was that time when all the food has been eaten, and all the bellies are full when the gathering of life finds the comfort of a story to close the night.

When the feast was finished, the people gathered around the fire, along with all of the animals that were there to be peaceful and warm and gentle in front of the fire.

Someone began to tell a story, as everyone covered themselves in warm blankets, full of food at the feast's end...

The storyteller gathered their voice and came to a spot by the fire, and in soft, gentle, soothing tones began to tell a story that would send everyone off into a dream, and the story went something like this...

Once upon a time, there was a place of greatest comfort.

And no matter where you are in this world, you can find it.

All you have to do is close your eyes, take a nice deep breath, and remember this place that you know in your heart.

It is the place where the feat is always being made, where the fire is always warm, where the friends are always close by to wrap you in their arms and soothe you into a loving slumber

This place is ancient and old, and yet it is fresh and new.

You have seen it in your dreams, and in your daytime, too.

It is everywhere and nowhere; it is always by your side.

It is within your very nature, this story of heart and mind.

This place of greatest comfort is the story you will tell every night when you go to sleep and find the place that suits you well.

This story is ongoing and will take you very far, deep into your dreamworld, to the farthest star.

Just gaze into the fire and hear the words unfold.

This is the place of greatest comfort, the greatest story ever told.

The whole world knows this story, for we all have it in our hearts to find our inner peace in a cottage safe at night.

All around the forest, deep to river's edge, down below the valley, in every cave, behind every rock, along the highest ledge, all the creatures are resting and feeling comfort under the night sky.

There is a community in the nighttime, and family of night.

There are always those around you, falling deeper into sleep- every animal, every bird, all of the people around you by the fire who hear the story in the place of greatest comfort.

The story drifts away from you as you ink deeper into relaxation and calm.

You have never felt so comfortable, so take care of, so whole.

The words from the story are faint and distant now.

You can hear it through your quiet mind as you breathe in deeply and feel the sublime joy of rest and comfort tonight.

You sink even more deeply into the blankets, and the cushions as the storyteller's voice becomes a part of your dream.

You are fully relaxed now and can let go of everything.

There is only this place for you now, this place of greatest comfort.

You are taken care of, loved, and held.

You are able to heal from this space, as you sleep, as you dream.

Your place of greatest comfort is always here for you and will always keep you safe and warm and protected as you trust your mind and body to fully release and relax, deep into your slumber.

Goodnight...sweet dreams...may your story continue tomorrow.

Chapter 5: Quiet Night in the Forest

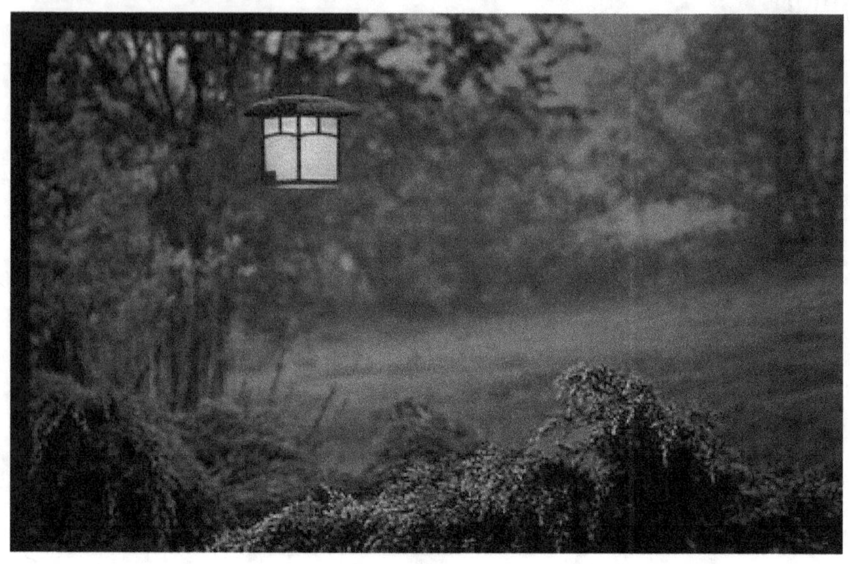

The moment you feel ready to take a journey into the forest at night, you will lay your body down and find comfort in the room where you are the calmest, most peaceful, and relaxed.

You will want to make sure that you are warm, covered with blankets, or wearing warm clothing.

Make your body feel as relaxed as possible so that you can go deeper into your thoughts and mind.

Finding your relaxed position, begin to breathe deeply. Notice your chest lifting, your abdomen extending.

Act upon the breath as slowly and steadily as you are able and hold for a count of one...two...three...release the breath as slowly and as steadily as you brought into your chest and body.

Again, with the feeling of total peace, pull oxygen into your chest and abdomen, filling the space within you as slowly and as steadily as you can...and hold the breath for a count of one...two...three...and release it as slowly as you pulled it into your body.

Your breathing can continue this way, or as it feels the most relaxing and calming to you.

Let your breath simply exist and do what it must to help you foster your serenity and sense of calm.

Your breath is pushing away any tension you may be feeling right now.

Your breath is helping you connect more fully to your body and your mind.

Your breath is sending you on a path of rest and rejuvenation.

Let your breath carry you there, quietly, slowly, steadily...

As you begin to sink into your mattress or cushions, wherever your body is laying down, you are going to begin to take a journey into the quiet of a forest at night, but first, you must get there.

The forest is not far.

It is a deeper part of you, a place inside of you that you are able to journey to when your body is at peace, and your breathing is relaxed.

Your inner world is made by you, and this quiet forest is a haven for you to become full of peaceful thoughts and empowered dreams to help you heal from the inside out.

Whatever you may be suffering from at this time in your life, sleeplessness, anxiety, worry...depression, frustration, self-doubt...whatever you are struggling with is going to be cleared in the quiet forest in the night.

All you have to do is find your way there from the comfort of this position you are laying in now.

You will get there easily: as your body becomes more relaxed through your breathing, as you allow yourself to let go of anything you might be clutching onto from the outside world, from your experiences, from your past...

Every breath will take you deeper into your relaxed body and state of mind.

You are here to travel into your subconscious mind and find a quiet space to release any fears, any doubts, your cares, and worries.

The quiet night in the forest is where you will go to heal these parts of you, these thoughts and feelings, these attitudes and beliefs...

The quiet of the forest realm will give you the permission and security you need to rest and dream without worry or grief.

All you have to do is relax more deeply into this position you are laying, your breath, relaxing into your deeper sense of self, falling deeper and deeper into the quiet night that surrounds you...

As you enter this space, you begin by noticing that your feet bare.

You look down and notice your bare feet standing on the ground.

The ground is safe and secure.

You feel comfortable here, with your feet bare, and you know that when you take a step forward, you will be walking towards your relief.

Your feet begin to carry you in that direction.

It is dark all around you, but for the silver moonlight that you can feel blanketing this landscape.

As you begin to notice what surrounds you in this space, you can feel the forest calling to you.

It is not far away, and you can see the shadow and silhouette of the trees and the ridge that the forest covers on the horizon...

Your bare feet are going to walk you forward toward that quiet forest.

It won't take long to get there.

It feels safe and familiar.

It feels welcoming and encouraging.

The quiet night in the forest is all that you need to feel at peace with your thoughts and your mind.

You can enjoy the relief that will come once you find your way through the forest to your place of total relaxation...

Your journey into this night forest has been a long time coming.

You have known this place before in your dreams from long ago.

It is an eternal forest that has always been a part of you.

It has always contained the peace of mind you are seeking.

In this forest, there is a hidden sanctuary of your truest self.

It is where you can feel whole in mind and spirit.

You enter the tree line of the woods and immediately feel a shift in the energy here.

It is so soothing and calm, so peaceful and serene.

You feel as though the trees are lovingly smiling upon you, welcoming you in with their girth and soft pine.

You can feel an energy of warmth radiating amongst all of the trees, plants, and other life here in the quiet forest.

There is nothing to run from here, nothing to hide from; there is only peace and comfort...

You hear a tinkling sound coming from somewhere distant, somewhere far off, deep in the wood.

You almost feel as if there are fairies and elves captivated by your presence in the forest.

You hear the sound again...it is calling you to follow it...

As you step all the way into the woods, you can see fireflies peppering the distant hills and groves within.

Their silent, quiet lights are friendly and guiding you forward on your path to the center of the quiet night in the forest.

They are everywhere, flashing warm, yellow-orange lights from their bodies, slowly dancing about the fresh, pine-scented forest...

You hear the soft tinkling again, and you begin to calmly follow it through the thickness of trees as the fireflies continue their merry dance of quiet light.

You follow the tinkling sound, like little bells or chimes being tickled by the night air of the wood.

There is a warmth to this sound, and you know that it is special and good, that it is guiding to just the right place...

You feel the soft, mossy earth beneath your feet, like a growing, velvet carpet that stretches out in every direction, comforting every footstep you take as you follow the tinkling bells further into the forest.

The only sound is the sound of your bare feet against the soft moss and the tinkling bell.

Everything else is soft, serene, gentle, and bathes in moonlight...

The forest is happy you are here, happy you have come.

It wants you to find peacefulness and relief.

The forest exists deep within you to offer you comfort from stress and worry relief from grief, and suffering.

The forest is here to hold your hand as you walk toward your destination of deep relaxation and a peaceful night's sleep...

Everywhere you look, you see glorious trees, fireflies, and the soft, pale moonlight touching everything it can.

You look ahead of you as the tinkling seems a little closer to you.

You feel a warmth and a glow from somewhere far away.

The distant glow asks you to come closer.

You know that it is safe and that there is friendliness in all parts of this quiet forest at night.

You can hear the tinkling bells more now.

The sound is coming from the warm glow at the center of a copse of trees, not too distant from where you are right now.

The fireflies are swimming through the air toward this place of light, and the bells are harmonious as they chime...

You find yourself close to the outside of the circle of trees and hiding behind one.

You look into the center of the warm and soothing glow.

At the center of the copse of trees is a beam of light, pouring out from the soil in a shaft or beam pointed up towards the starlight.

You cannot tell if the beam of light is coming from the cosmos and the stars, or from the warm center of the Earth...

Above the beam of light, high up in the trees, you notice a treehouse.

You see a set of steps to climb up to the treehouse.

At the top of the tree it is sitting in, and you notice a small set of wind chimes dangling from the treehouse roof.

There is the sound that I called you to this center.

There is the sacred space that has been calling out you since you entered the forest...

Coming out from behind the tree, you enter the copse and walk toward the shaft of light glowing from the center and beaming up to the heavens through past the treehouse.

You are here to resolve all of your tension and stress, all of your anxiety and worry and doubt.

This circle of trees, this shaft of light, this is where you cleanse yourself of all of the thoughts and emotions that keep you feeling far away from rest, that keeps you locked in cycles of doubt and worry.

You will now step forward into the beam of light and allow yourself to be bathed in it.

This light is coming from high above from the cosmic life flow of the distant planets and stars.

This light is coming from deep within the Earth.

It is all connected, going up and down all at once.

And now, as you are stepping into this light, you are able to feel the total purity of mind and spirit that comes from true relief...

You have all that you need right here, right now, in this beam of light.

You have everything you will need to find peace of mind and body and get the rest that you deserve.

You no longer have to carry any burdens or fears.

You can release them into this beam of light and let them return to the cosmic flow of all things.

This light is here to take your pain and suffering and return it to the life force of the Universe, transforming into something else, something more positive for you...

Stand in this beam of light in the circle of trees in the quiet night in the forest.

Feel yourself releasing all of your grief and anxiety, all of your frustration, all of your negative thoughts and ideas, into this warm and healing beam of light, this light that flows freely from one source to another...

You can give all of your painful memories, your traumas, your wounds, and hurts to this light.

It will take care of that energy for you.

You can give it what ails you, depresses you, keeps you feeling afraid at night, all of that can go directly into this beam of light.

As you stand here, feel this warm glowing beam flow through the soles of your bare feet, up through your ankles and your legs.

See and feel this light go through your knees and thighs, up through your hips and pelvis...

Follow this light up through your torso, filling your abdomen, your organs, your bloodstream.

See the shaft of light going into your arms and hands, your chest, neck, shoulders.

See the light filling your headspace.

Now see the light coming from above going down through your body, circulating through all the way out of your feet and into the Earth.

Feel the light passing in both directions through your body, from the crown of your head through your limbs, through your feet, into the soil, down...down...down to the Earth's core...

This light is a part of you, and you are a part of it—it is the cosmic lifeforce of both Earth and Stars, and it is here to relieve you of your doubts and fears.

You are alone in this light in this circle of trees, and all you have to do is breathe and watch it fill your whole being with soft comfort and powerful awakening...

You are letting go now of all of the worries and cares of your mind.

You are refreshing your powerful inner light, your true sense of self, your deeper intuition, and sense of knowing that everything will be alright and that all you have to do right now is breathe, relax and let your whole being become full of this light...

You can see the light reflecting off of the trees that are encircling you.

They are wise, old, and powerful.

They are full of healing light and energy and will continue to hold you and keep you safe in the quiet night in the forest.

When you are ready, you notice the steps that will lead you to the treetop and into the treehouse.

Full of light, you decide to climb up to the top and into the warm and welcoming home high up in the trees...

As you climb, you can look down and see the glowing shaft of light remains available to you whenever you need to release any negative thoughts or energies from your body and your mind.

It will always remain here in this quiet forest in the night, here for you whenever you need it...

The glow of the beam of light reflects off of the treehouse, and as you climb up to the balcony, you notice the chimes that were blowing in the soft night breeze, ringing out to you, calling you to this copse of trees and this place of light.

You reach your hand out and give them a jingle...

Climbing inside of the treehouse, you see that it is safe and warm and has all that you need to get a good night's rest.

Here, high up in the forest at night, you are full of light and loving energy from the Earth and the Stars.

You are free of all of your pain and worry, all of your anxiety and stress.

This treehouse is made up of just the way you like it and will give you a soothing place to lay down and rest your head, welcoming you into the dreams that await you...

As you lay down and pull a pillow under your head, you see a firefly float into the treehouse and glow a few times as it passes by your pillow.

You are safe and warm and serene.

The forest of trees is guarding you as you rest in the treehouse high up off the ground.

The fireflies gather around, lighting up the forest throughout the night...

You take another deep breath in and let yourself fall fast...asleep...

Chapter 6: A Trip into Starlight

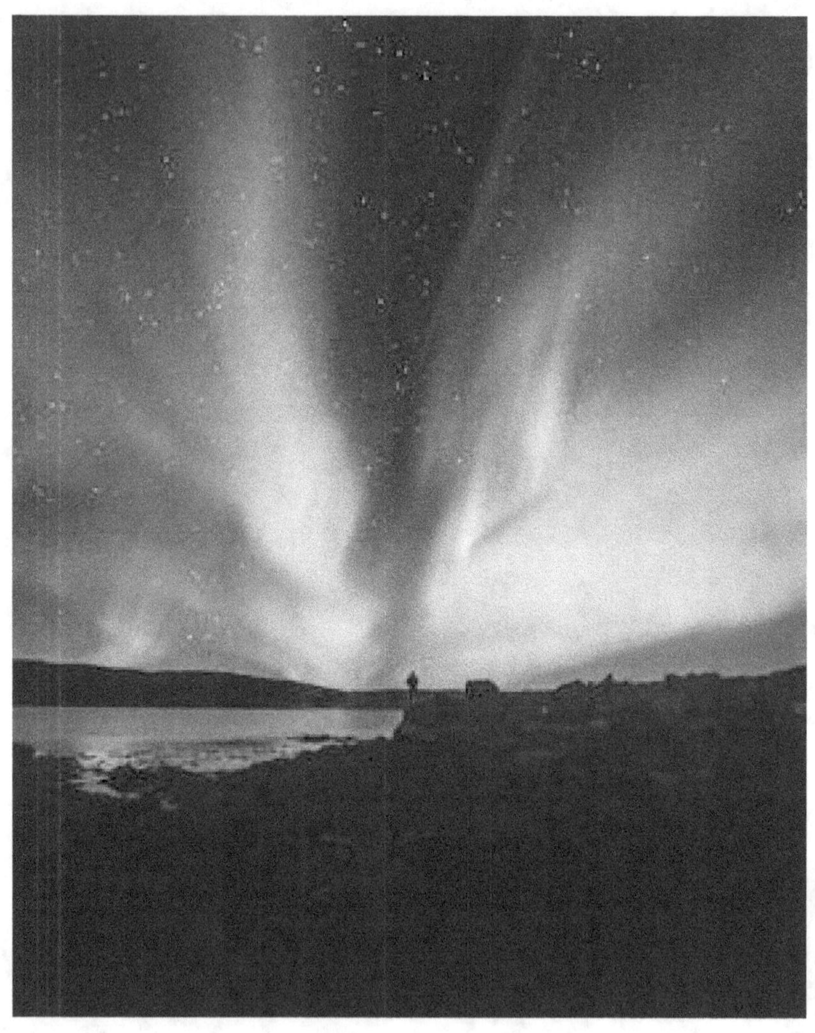

The night sky holds many wonders and distant mysteries.

For ages, we had gazed up at the stars and looked for answers to our deepest questions, for have used the maps made by the stars to carry us home, and we had told many tales about when mortals became legend, forever twinkling in the night.

As you prepare for your long journey into dreams and the unconscious, you will find yourself carried to these distant shores far from your life on Earth and amidst some of the most glorious visions, you can imagine...

Turn off the world around you and prepare to take a journey off the planet and into the cosmic starlight beyond. Ask your body to find the most comfortable position.

Lean into that position and scan your whole body for any tension, aches, and pains, anything you might be holding onto physically.

Find those spaces and consciously release them.

Let it all go with your breath.

Relaxation begins with your breath, and throughout this meditation bedtime story, keeping a steady breath will help you find a fully relaxed body, mind, and heart.

You can begin with your breath by simply drawing it into your nostrils and exhaling it out of your nostrils or mouth.

Breathe in slowly, exhale slowly.

Inhale...exhale...

Your sense of calm, your serenity, your peace of mind, lives in your breath.

Allow it to continue as you allow your body to fully release all of the tension you are still carrying from your day, your week, even the past several months.

Feel it vacate your body and let all of your muscles turn to jam or jelly.

If your muscles feel hard, soften them.

If your muscles feel tight, loosen them.

Use your breath to find this physical sensation...

Your body is now longer, smoother energy, your muscles are letting go of all of your current stress, and you are now a little more relaxed than you were before.

All of your breathing throughout these moments has taken you farther into your peacefulness and calmness.

All of your inhales and exhales have loosened your grip on the day...

Now that you are a little more relaxed, you can begin to go on your bigger journey into relief and healing.

Your journey begins when you step out of your house.

In your mind, see yourself walking outside of your house and into the night.

You are safe and warm, and you are now standing outside of your house under the starry night sky...

The stars are bright.

There are no lights around you.

It is totally black outside except for the starlight.

You feel enveloped by starlight as you look up and see it stretching from one horizon to the other.

The stars are endless, and there isn't a cloud in the sky.

It is clear, and you can see all of the stars in your hemisphere...

Continuing your breath, you welcome the starlight into you as you breathe in, breathing in the feeling of connection to the great unknown, the distant mysteries of the far-off galaxies beyond.

This starlight fills your whole body with each breath and invites you to take a trip to a far-off distant place, somewhere deep within the cosmos...

There is nothing to fear, for you are here to journey.

Your physical body will not be harmed by going so far away.

You can see your journey through the vastness of your inner mind.

There are places you will go to that you will never journey with your physical body, but tonight, you can fly.

Tonight you are free to float away and ascend into the highest reaches of starlight...

You feel your body become weightless as you begin to lift off of the surface of the Earth.

You are not afraid to fly.

It is as if you have always known how to fly and to float in this way.

It feels natural and good.

You let your body lift from this place you were standing, and as you get higher off the ground, you feel yourself being pulled higher and higher up into the dark night of stars...

When you look down, you know you will not fall.

You are in control of your flight, and you have always flown like this.

It is easy to do, and you are relaxed as you take off.

When you look down, you watch the Earth begin to diminish.

The farther you go up to the stars, the smaller the buildings become, the cars, the trains, the highways, the rivers, mountains, and streams...all are becoming smaller and farther away, more distant...

You are falling up...up...up...into the starry night where there is nothing but you and the light of each star twinkling at you.

When you look behind you, Earth is far away, and you are closer to the moon now.

The moon is welcoming and bright. It feels small compared to the Earth you just came from. It is big enough for you to sit upon...

You connect to the surface of the moon, and you sit down with your eyes pointing back at the Earth.

You feel as if you can see everything more clearly now.

You are far away from your problems, your cares, and worries and you can see your life from the outside looking in—you can feel how different it is to look at yourself and your life from this perspective...

Here on the moon, you feel open and happy that you can look back at the Earth in this way and reflect.

You can contemplate here and find answers to solve your problems and challenges.

You can see clearly from here because you are not right in it—you are closer to yourself at this moment.

You are closer to your higher purpose when you come to this place of stillness deep within...

From here on the moon, you feel the brightness of the sun reflecting off of the surface.

The silvery moonlight feels like it is wrapping itself around you, like an ethereal blanket of security and comfort.

The luminosity is recharging your batteries and helping you to feel rejuvenated and refreshed, like bathing in light...

Your breath comes in, and you can breathe easily here.

You are of the cosmos and so you can survive in this place.

You are ready to carry on and go deeper into the calming serenity of Universal light.

You are going where no one can go on Earth, and you are going there with your thoughts, with your subconscious, with your intuition guiding you...

You are going to get ready to leave the moon and travel even farther beyond.

As you stand up on the surface, you feel your body bend at the knees and then push you off the surface.

You begin to float out, away from the moon, being pulled forward into the starry night, beyond Earth, beyond the moon, beyond time...

You can feel yourself getting farther and farther away, and you feel serene, safe, and in control.

You are the captain of this interstellar flight.

You are safe and your body is capable of taking this trip.

You are here to find your cosmic truth.

You are here to set yourself free.

You can see your entire reality so clearly from all the way out here, far off into the starry night.

You are here to be, to exist, to enjoy the freedom that exists here.

You are burdened by nothing.

You have no obligations here.

You have only your inner power, your truth, your release from all of your current life problems, and challenges.

You are safe to leave all of your cares and worries in the vastness of the cosmos, in the deep of outer space...

You are free to realize your deepest truth in this place in space.

You are open to all things, and it feels safe and calm.

This is a calm, centered really.

The starlight is holding you closely, protecting you on your journey into the distant realms of space.

You are entering a space that is colorful and big.

A nebula is forming in front of your eyes, like a cosmic waterfall of blue and gold dust speckled with red and green starlight.

This starry cloud of dust opens to you like flower petals blooming on a rose.

You are invited to come closer to it and let yourself fall through it, like a tunnel into another reality.

Getting closer and closer to this massive, smoky, rainbow, you begin to feel pulled into it softly.

It is gentle and calm, and you are not in a hurry, out here in the great beyond...

The nebula surrounds you softly, gently.

It begins to turn into a tunnel that your body can float through.

You are not sure where the tunnel will lead, but you are calm and relaxed.

You don't need to know.

You are full of the power of the cosmos, and you are at peace in your mind and your body.

You allow your body to just glide through the nebula tunnel, feeling open to whatever lies beyond...

You are transported through the tunnel until you feel your body sitting on a sandy shore...you take a look around at this space, a wide, vast landscape on another planet, somewhere in a distant galaxy.

You can feel the softness of the sand.

It is different from Earth's sand, softer, finer, blue-green in places, and splotches of yellow and red in others...

The air is fresh here.

You can breathe easily.

You feel relaxed and calm, curiously taking in the place you have found through the tunnel.

You can feel the air is warm but not too hot.

You can feel a soft breeze that brings you into contact with a beautiful scent on the air.

There are strange and exotic flowers and plants that look foreign, alien to you.

You are drawn to their unique qualities and colors, like nothing you have ever seen on Earth before...

Sitting here in this place, you are able to feel the calmness of your mind, body, and heart.

You are in total peace and centeredness.

You are far away and in a place where you are safe to rest and relax.

The landscape that you have found is comforting and pleasant, and as you lay back on the softest sand, you look up into the starry night sky.

You can see the galaxy far, far away that you traveled from, and you know that you will be resting there in your home when it is time to go back.

You are ready to leave the soft sand of this other world and begin your return flight home.

You stand up and take a deep breath in, pulling in all of the wonderful serenity of this far-off distant shore.

The nebula gas returns and pulls you in, as if it never left you, as if it was always there, waiting for you to return home...

You are ready to transcend space and time once more and travel back through the tunnel.

You find your way through the nebula tunnel with ease and grace, moving slowly, gently.

You are drawing closer and closer to the space where you entered the tunnel, and as you come out of it, you find yourself back in the vastness of outer space, covered in starlight.

You are pulled from the nebula, floating back through the cosmos the way that you came, retracing your steps through the ethereal realms of the stars.

Each breath you take in and exhale will push you forward to your destination.

Each inhale gives you the life force you need to propel yourself back home.

Each exhale gets you closer to your healing and relief, letting it all go and leaving it way out here in space...

You are much closer to home now because you can see the moon again.

You are narrowing in on the moon, and you decide to take a break here before making the final trip home to your house.

You float toward the surface of the moon and gracefully land, finding a comfortable spot to sit and absorb the luminosity of the moon's surface.

You have all of the time in the universe to just sit here and relax for a moment...

Sitting here, looking at the Earth from the moon, you recognize your home.

From far away, you can relate to everything and everyone.

You can feel the earnest efforts of all people to lead a good life and search for a deeper truth.

Looking out upon the Earth from this place, you remind yourself that even the biggest problems you face are little compared to the energy of all life in the Universe.

Here you can feel refreshed, relaxed, the calm of mind and body.

You are everything and everyone, everywhere, right in this moment of reflection, all the way out here on the Moon, surrounded by stars.

As you ponder the significance of your life and the life of all others down there on Earth, let your breath continue to be slow and steady, filling you with gratitude and acceptance, letting in forgiveness and trust, patience and compassion...

When you are ready to return, you can float back to the Earth and enter your deepest comfort and rest.

You stand up on the moon's surface and prepare to launch.

You push yourself off of the surface and glide slowly and peacefully toward the Earth.

You are following the same path you took to get up to the stars.

It will take you right back to your house, where you stood outside and looked up at the starlight...

You are getting closer and closer to the Earth's surface, and the moon is a distant friend again.

You can feel yourself being pulled in the right direction.

You are not in a hurry.

You are not picking up speed.

You are gently floating, flying home slowly, delicately, peacefully.

The mountains and trees, the rivers and streams are beginning to become larger, closer, as you slowly descend back to the surface of your home planet.

You are closer now, and all of the buildings and cars, buses, and people are coming closer and clearer into view.

Your body is slow and steady, like a hot air balloon, floating quietly and calmly to the ground.

As you get closer to your home, you are ready to land.

You touch the surface of the Earth with your toe, followed by your foot, and then your other foot lands, and you are now two feet back on the ground, back on Earth...

You turn your head to look back up at the starry night sky.

You are home again, and that was also your home for a time.

You let go of all of your worries and cares up there, and you are now ready to walk back inside of your house and find yourself ready to fall fast asleep...

You go inside, close the door, walk to your room where you are laying down, and go deeper...and deeper...and deeper into sleep...

Chapter 7: The Ship and the Sea

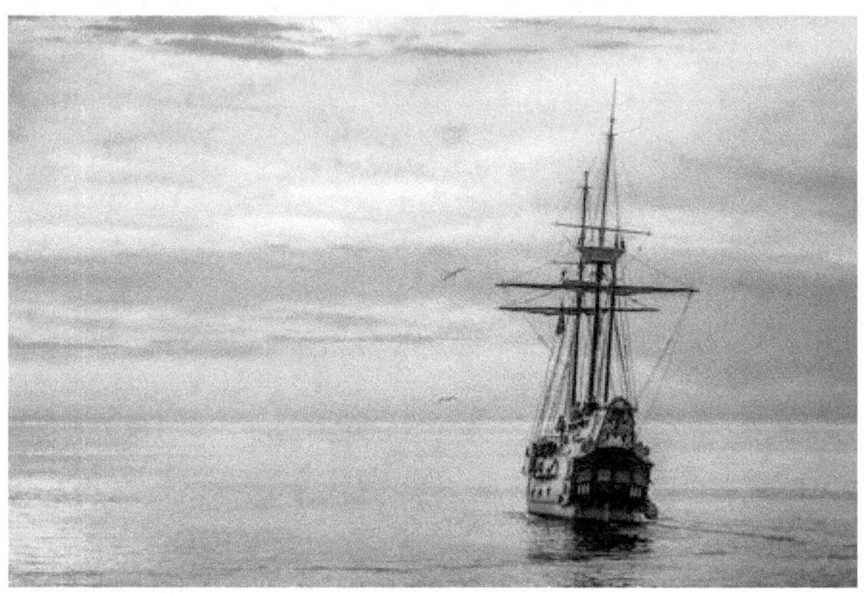

You are on your way to a sacred island, and the only way there is by ship.

Your journey will take time and feel soothing as you connect to the rhythm and embrace of the ocean waves.

You will begin your journey through your breath.

Your breath will help you release anything you may be holding onto at this time—anything from your day, your week...

You will start to feel your body relaxing more as you inhale and exhale, letting all of your cares and worries slip away from you.

Wherever you find tension in your body, let it release with your breath out.

Every breath lets you sink further into relaxation and comfort.

Inhale deeply, pulling fresh air into your muscles, your joints, and bones, your ligaments.

Inhale into your organs and tissues.

Exhale any discomforts you may be holding onto.

Let them naturally relax out of you with your breath.

Enjoy the change in your body as you grow more relaxed with each new, refreshing breath cycle.

You will begin to feel heavier, sinking into your mattress or cushions more and more.

At the same time, you will feel lighter and freer, unshackled from pain and tension, anxiety, and stress...

Let your relief spill over and fill the room that surrounds you.

Let the energy of your peacefulness resonate and radiate into the atmosphere.

As you become lighter and freer, the heavier and more relaxed your body feels.

Fill the room with your serene position.

Begin to feel the surrounding room take a new shape and form as you continue your breath...

You are on a warm beach.

You hear a flock of seagulls cawing in the distance.

You can hear the constant churning of the sea, the waves rolling luxuriously over themselves, breaking into white foam on the wet shore.

You are laying in the sand, and it feels perfectly warm on your body.

The sand is soft and dry where you are, and you are soothed by the temperature and the texture of the sand as you listen to the white-noise rhythm of the sea...

Here on this beach, you are perfectly still.

The sun's rays are at just the right temperature to feel relaxing and healing.

The light behind your eyelids is a soft, warm peachy-orange hue, from the sunlight hitting the skin of your face.

You can feel the hairs on your arm wave quietly in a gentle breeze, sending refreshing vibrations through your body...

The ocean is endless and vast.

You can feel its majesty from where you are laying, several meters away from the rolling surf.

The passion of the roaring sea is calling to you, asking you to traverse it with your courage and your love of adventure.

You sit up and look around at the beach, the shore, the twinkling diamond-light that shimmers on the water's surface...

On the horizon, you see a ship.

This ship is made of iron and wood.

It is the ship that has carried you far in life.

It has taken you everywhere you have wanted or needed to go.

This ship is, here again, to take you forward on your path of inner healing and relief.

You will find yourself feeling very drawn to this ship, feeling the urge to climb back on board, and take your next journey to heal the soul...

Standing up, you walk across the sand and feel it transform under your feet: from soft and dry, to damp, to wet as you get closer to the ocean waves.

Standing barefoot on this soothing wet sand, you wait for the tide to return and wrap around your ankles.

As the seawater pushes toward you, you feel a rise in your excitement, anticipating the feeling of water cresting your skin...

As the waves curl around your ankles and feet, you notice how warm the water feels.

It is soothing, warm, refreshing, and clear.

It feels powerful against your skin and helps you to feel alive to your deeper truth and inner knowing.

You have all of your worries and cares to let go of and the water in the waves begins to absorb all of the negative thoughts or feelings that you carry with you...

You are able to feel refreshed now, as the tide pulls away from you like a steady exhale from your lungs.

The tide takes away any feelings that you have right now that you want to let go of and release.

As the water pulls out and away, ebbing as an exhale, another flowing wave is coming back in to wash away any of your feelings of uncertainty or fear, any feelings of concern or worry...

Your feeling lighter and freer.

Your body is warm and relaxed in the sun and the water.

You are being relieved of your stress here at this moment.

Connect to your breath along with the ocean tide in your mind and let go of what wants to be set free and released...

You are ready to follow your journey forward now.

You are ready to make your journey to the ship so that you can set sail and find your deepest relaxation.

The ship is a great distance from you, and you will have to find your way there.

You are able to grow a fishtail and swim.

When you enter the seawater fully, you give your body to the energy of the ocean and of the water…

You become like a merman or merwoman, a human fish who swims with the dolphins and whales and finds great comfort in the warm, salty surface of the water.

Stepping fully into the water, you feel your tail form and propel you forward.

You are swimming close to the surface to feel the sun's rays on your body.

You can see the diamond twinkle of the sun reflecting on the water as you gain speed with your fins…

You feel the water gliding across your skin.

You are able to easily roll around in the water like a dolphin or a seal, playfully swimming and streaking through the water with joy.

Your body feels smooth and alive, fresh and clean as you go through the water, gaining speed and feeling light as air.

As you continue your trajectory toward the ship, you notice a pod of dolphins to either side of you as you swim.

They are jumping out of the water and arching through the air by your side, encouraging your journey forward, cheering you on as they swim alongside you.

They are with you all the way to your ship, your protectors in the sea, your escorts in the water…

You are nearing your ship, and as you get closer, you begin to realize just how massive it is.

This is the boat of your inner mind that takes you through your thoughts and dreams, your emotions, and your beliefs.

This ship helps you find your path, your goals, your fantasies, and your desires.

This ship was made for you alone, and only you can steer the helm…

The ship is now within your grasp.

You swim right up to the side and note how ancient it looks, like an old-world cargo, or pirate ship, back in the days when you only used stars to find your way home…

It has seen many trips to many shores, and tonight is another journey.

You find a foothold and a ladder that leads up the side of the ship.

You are able to climb aboard this way, your fins and tail turning back into your regular limbs, lifting you up the ladder, one step at a time…

You are climbing over the rail and find yourself on deck.

You are the only one on board—the captain and the crew, and you only need yourself to take this journey.

You find your way to the helm of the ship so that you may steer it on course.

Where is your course going to take you?

Where does this ocean adventure lead?

With your hands gripping the wheel at the helm, you decide in your thoughts that you are ready to move forward.

Just as you think this thought, the ship pushes forward, slowly getting a move on, as if your thoughts were the wind that blew the sails.

You are in motion now.

Your ship is moving forward...

You are going farther out to sea now, where there is no land, where there is no one.

It is just you and the rocking ship of your dream world.

You can feel the wind lift the sails and put a breeze in your hair.

The sun is shining as you get farther from the shore.

You can look back now and see the spot on the beach where you were first beginning this journey.

You can see where you swam with the dolphins disappearing behind you as you steer further out.

The horizon is long and ageless.

It reaches out in all directions, curving around the Earth.

You are free here.

Alone, but not afraid.

Alone but not lonely.

Alone but full of love and light for your own path.

You are now surrounded by the ocean.

You are far out to sea, and the wind has pushed your ship far forward into serenity, peace, and calm.

Your feelings are free to expand here.

There is enough space for all of your thoughts and feelings, for all of your dreams and passions, for all of your intentions and needs...

This vast watery landscape holds the key to your openness with yourself.

Underneath the surface is all of your hidden truths.

You are going to find them slowly over time as you explore the realms of your unconscious on your ship of dreams.

There is nothing more sacred than to be at peace within yourself.

The waters of this ocean that you are sailing on are the waters of yourself.

You have nothing to hide or fear from yourself.

Everything that appears to you here that comes up for healing in this place is going to help you find your deeper truth, your deeper self-knowing, your relief...

Your ship is slowing now, and it is time to let the sails lay low as you are set adrift on the wide, open sea.

The breeze brings rhythm to the water's edge.

You feel that rhythm in the rocking of the ship, steady, long, slow, back and forth, bobbing grandly in the sun.

It is a comforting rhythm.

It is subtle and deep.

It is the vibration of light on water, with air from the wind and fire from the sun.

You are here to heal and renew.

You are here to refresh, and here the ocean revives your soul.

You can feel yourself being soothed by the rocking of the ship.

You listen to the water lapping up against the side of the ship, the sound of water on wood...

You feel focused, serene, peaceful.

You are free to just sit on the deck and watch the sunbeams turn into bright pinks and oranges, purples and lavenders, as the sun starts its descent into the water.

The bright red-orange sun becomes hot pink as it smears against the water's surface.

The water is colored now with the light of the setting sun...

You are here, reflecting the opening of your soul in this water.

This water waves with the frequency of your mind and your thoughts.

The gentle ripple of the ocean reflects your peacefulness and calmness.

You are as the water, ebbing and flowing, rocking and swaying, soothing and refreshing...

The power of this water fills your soul and lets you feel connected to your primal roots, your ancient wisdom, your sacred intuition.

The waterline is thick against the sides of your ship.

You feel perfectly safe and calm as the sun sizzles into the western horizon, and the stars come out to shine through the night...

In the soothing ocean night, you feel held by the quiet and peace of this place.

You are far away, listening to the water, hearing nothing but your own rhythm on the sea.

You feel embraced by your own journey and adventure into the deep unknown.

You feel refreshed to have all that you are right inside of you...always...

You feel the starlight on your skin.

They are the only lights for hundreds of miles in all directions.

You look up at the stars and then down at the ocean water.

There is a perfect, crystal clear reflection of the starry night sky on the surface of the water. As far as the eye can see, in all directions, from horizon to horizon, above and below, there are stars.

The stars of the water are a mirror image of the stars in the sky.

It is like floating through a sea of stars, like floating through space, far from the surface of the Earth...

You feel like you have been here before, in this starry expanse, like you could really be floating far out in the cosmos.

Then, you hear the lapping of the water, and you remember your ship is with you, holding you, taking you forward on your journey, and wherever it is going to lead you, far off in your dreams and sleep...

The starlight surrounding you, from the sky and the water below, fill your heart and mind with soothing relief.

You are safe and content to just be here on the deck of this ship.

The air is warm.

The rhythm of the ship is rocking you gently, back and forth...back and forth...back and forth...

You are at peace now, in your body, in your mind, in your heart.

You have all that you need to feel at ease, far away in the starry night of the ocean.

Your ship is carrying you to your dreams now, and you can feel the boat push forward, wind, in the sails as you lay in comfort on the deck under the stars.

Your ship knows where to go and will deliver you to your dreamscape as you sail farther and farther off into the horizon...

Your dreams will come as the sun rises in the East.

You will begin to find the place in your subconscious thoughts where your ship of dreams wants to take you tonight.

You will find everything you need there.

All you have to do now is just rest here.

Let your ship take you forward.

Let the soothing sway of the boat rock you gently on your journey tonight...

Feel the light of the stars turning pink with morning's promise as you drift farther and farther into dreamland...

Your ship will carry you there...just breathe.

Chapter 8: Animal Dreams

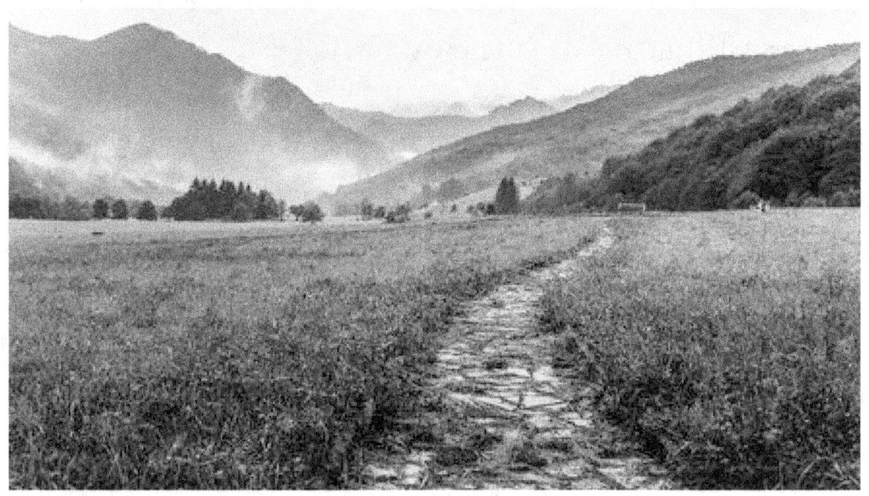

In every good fable, you will find an animal that helps to tell a story.

In every place in nature, you find the whimsical and ethereal beasts who call Mother Earth home, just like you.

For centuries, many different peoples have looked to animals for messages of truth, divination, omens of things to come, and ways to feel protected, brave, and safe.

Your personal spirit animal may not be the same every time you meditate on them.

Sometimes, an animal spirit guide will come to you to help foster growth and change in new ways.

All animals are symbolic of something, and all of your experiences with this mediation will give you the messages that you need right now on your path.

Look to the animal spirits for their symbolic messages and what they might represent to you as you go on your meditation journey.

Ask your animal spirit guide to come to you through your dreams to show you a path that is just right for you...right now.

You may have the same spirit animal come to you many times, or you may meet a variety of animal spirit guides on your path.

For whatever reason, the animal that comes to you today is the one with the answers for your journey.

You can find friendship and take comfort in your animal guides and learn from them what magic awaits you when you enter into an animal dream.

For this guided meditation, find a comfortable and relaxing position to enjoy as you relax your body and mind.

You can lay on the floor, in your bed, on some cushions...anywhere that feels safe, relaxing, and calming.

You may want to fall asleep, and that's okay.

Your animal will still come and find you when the time is right...in your dreams...on a walk in nature...

You are going to find your relief through a walk through the kingdom of animals.

To begin, find your inhale.

Relax into yourself as you breathe in deeply and let go of your day or your week as you let your breath out. Inhale slowly, relaxing into your body a little further...and exhale away the last few hours, days, weeks...anything that is in need of release...

Inhale gently, slowly...give your body all of the fresh air it needs to feel refreshed and relieved...exhale slowly, steadily, letting out the tension and stress of life, giving yourself permission to simply let go and relax.

Continue your breathing in this way for several breath cycles...

You are more relaxed now.

You have a heaviness to your muscles because you know you don't need to go anywhere or do anything.

You are exactly where you need to be right now, and you will not have to get up anytime soon.

Let go of any worries and cares that you should be accomplishing something else right now.

Your only purpose at this time is rest and relaxation.

You can wander freely in the animal kingdom from this place of true relaxation.

Your body and your mind are free to go on a journey to a long-forgotten land where the elders whispered stories of the great beasts and birds of legend, the ones who told the tales of strength and courage, of tenderness and patience, of dedication or perseverance...

The animals of the ancient world are similar to the ones you see walking around today.

In the landscape of your mind, on your journey into deeper awareness, your animal spirit guide can resemble anything at all...any color...any size...any shape...any texture.

Your dream animal is your companion into the dream world, who will lead you toward a sense of trust with yourself and the power you hold within.

As you inhale again, breathe into a distant place...a landscape far off in your dreamland.

Look around this place and notice what it looks like.

What are the features you notice?

Is it a desert, a lake, a forest?

Are you on an island covered in jungle, or in a tropical rainforest?

Are you somewhere near the ocean?

Explore your landscape in your mind for a moment and let yourself wander through this hidden realm of your subconscious mind...

Take a few deep breaths and really open yourself to the feeling of this space.

What does the ground below your feet feel like?

How hot or cold is it? Is it cloudy and raining, or warm and sunny?

Do you feel a breeze or a strong wind?

Focus on the details of your landscape.

Allow it to truly come to life for you in your mind…

As you feel yourself becoming more relaxed and in tune with your inner world, you notice a path.

The path is made for you to follow it.

The path is leading you closer to your destination and your animal guide.

For some, your animal guide may have already shown up for you, and that's okay.

The animal guide will still ask you to walk this path, and it will walk with you…

If you have not seen the animal come forward for you yet, do not struggle to make it appear.

It will come to you when you are in the right moment of relaxation and relief.

You will now begin to walk on this path, one step at a time.

Use your imagination to give life to the world you have created in your mind.

You are an explorer, and you have the power to imagine the detail of this place as you walk through it.

The path is not straight. It winds and bends and takes you over and under, out and through, around and behind.

It circles through this landscape in ways only you can see.

You will continue to walk this path and follow it through, taking note of the surroundings of your mind...

The path is beginning to level out now, and it has become straight and pointing straight ahead into a thick fog.

The fog has come out of nowhere, but it is where your path is taking you.

You will need to continue walking on the path through the fog.

As you enter this thick, moist haze, the world around you becomes softer, blurred, distant...

The fog is enshrouding you and making it hard for you to see clearly what is on the other side, and yet, you know that you must continue forward and make this journey further along on your path.

You are being guided to your spirit animal who is waiting for you on the other side, to come together with you and help you find peace and calm from within...

You are getting closer now, but you are not afraid.

You know that the creatures of this world are not harmful.

They are here to keep you safe and help you find a deeper path and greater truth.

They are here to inspire you and make you feel relieved to have a friend.

You are getting more excited, thinking about what animal may be arriving to act as your guide in the dreamworld tonight...

Let the path pull you forward through the fog. Inhale deeply...and exhale slowly, preparing yourself to meet your animal friend.

Your journey will begin again once you have encountered this creature.

You feel yourself getting nearer as the fog begins to lift, and you can see more clearly.

As the smoke clears, relax, and just look.

Don't tell yourself what it is going to be; just see it.

There on the path in front of you, right now, is your animal spirit guide who will escort you on your journey.

The fog is fully lifted, and the animal is here before you, awaiting you on the road.

Take a few moments to observe your animal friend.

Let them take shape.

See the details of their shape, form, texture, and size.

Notice what kind of fur or feather or scales they might have.

Notice the shape of their eyes, their nose, their mouth.

Do they have whiskers?

A beak?

A snout?

Show yourself fully what your animal spirit guide looks like and let the vision of their shape sit with you for a moment before you move forward...

The animal that has come to you, no matter whether it is snake or bear, octopus or hummingbird, squirrel or pigeon, it will have an important message for you as you drift further off into sleep and find your deepest comfort.

The wisdom of your animal guide is strong and old.

It will know how to help you find what you are looking for in this place...

Let the animal come closer to you and make contact.

It will not hurt you or run away in fear.

This animal has come to you on purpose, to connect with you and help you along the road.

Feel it, sense its energy with your inner mind.

Show yourself how it feels to be closer to this creature in your imagination...

As you bond with your animal companion, give them an opportunity to show you a message.

Anything that they do could be helpful for you, and it is up to you to interpret what that message is.

Don't overthink it.

Just let it come to you naturally.

It might not come until tomorrow or a few days from now, and that's okay.

You may need time to reflect on the mystical purpose of your animal guide...

Continue to inhale deeply, relaxing into this moment, into feeling out the power of your animal guide.

Allow that essence or spirit to circulate within and around you.

Let this being give you the opportunity to see something more clearly, to direct your focus in a new way, to take comfort in a hidden answer to a long-asked question…

You will begin to feel the opening of your gift from this animal guide as you continue forward into your dreams tonight.

For now, you can continue to travel through your mindscape with your new friend.

Let the animal pick which way you are going to go, and follow.

See what direction the creature will take and trust that they have your best interests at heart.

They are here to help you find what you are looking for…

The path is long and winding, and perhaps your guide has taken you off the beaten track and into other subconscious realms.

There is no wrong path.

Your guide knows where to take you, and you can trust them to keep you safe and secure.

Your guide is leading you into new territory, a place you have never been or seen in your mind before.

You are close together; they never stray too far from your side.

This creature has gotten you closer to something you value, something of great importance to you in your life.

You can feel that there is something opening inside of you, something that you have needed to be shown by a trusted friend and guide...

Your animal guide is letting you know with their own energy and actions that you need to stop on the path and wait.

They want you to listen to your heart for a few moments so that you are ready to see what they have wanted to show you.

As you inhale and exhale for a few breath cycles, connect to your heart center.

Breathe into your soul, your mind, your body.

Let the breath fill you with warmth and compassion for your own unique life story...

The animal wants you to see what comes next on your path.

Your guide wants to show you what you need to be thinking about, focusing on, realizing.

They are asking you to stand tall and connect to yourself fully so that you can look even deeper into your heart for answers...for the truth...

Your animal guide is giving you strength while you are paused here, giving you comfort and relief, becoming an even closer friend and ally by supporting your journey.

They are ready to help you forward now.

You are back on the footpath, and the fog has returned.

You can hardly see through it, but your animal guide is with you now, leading you forward.

You have nothing to fear...

Your guide disappears into the fog as you continue to slowly walk the path.

You feel and see the fog lifting now, and your animal friend is waiting for you here, guarding a sacred doorway that leads to your heart center.

What is behind this door is what your heart desires most right now.

Let this knowledge come to you without worry, or fear, or regret...

Feel grateful that you are here to grow and that you are being guided and shown the path that will help you the most.

Honor and trust that no matter what is on the other side of this door, you will always be loved, protected, and safe with your animal guide...

You step forward to the door in the middle of the path that seems to lead into nothing and nowhere.

You lay your hand on the knob and turn it.

Your animal guide is by your side and can help you find your way through.

The door is open now.

See what is on the other side.

You may not be ready to step through the doorway yet, but you are certainly welcome to just look within and discover your truth.

Stand tall with your animal guide beside you and let yourself look deep within your heart...your mind...your soul.

This is what your friend wanted to show you.

This is what you are being guided to see.

Take it in as you take in another few breaths in and out.

Spend time noticing what this means to you.

When you are ready, you can step through the doorway with your animal companion by your side.

Let them guide you further now into the world of dreams.

Let them show you where the path leads from here...

You are not alone.

You are safe to be whatever you need to be right now through the wisdom of this creature and friend.

Open your mind to your dream state and let yourself be carried into the depths of your mysterious and otherworldly unconscious mind.

Your animal spirit guide is here to guard you and keep you safe.

You are protected.

You are able to just rest now, knowing that they will take care of you all night long, no matter where your journey will lead you.

Take another deep breath in and sigh it out.

It is time to dream, and your animal guide will see you through...all the way 'til morning....

Chapter 9: The Hot Air Balloon Ride

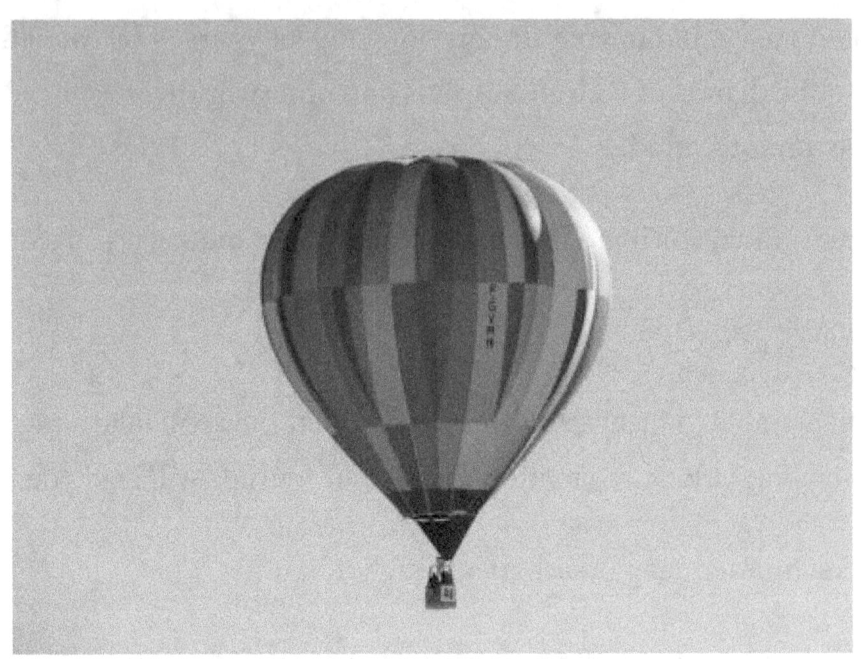

Sometimes, all you need is to feel far from all of your cares and worries.

Sometimes, all you need is to glide through life on a serene cloud, floating across a pale blue sky.

If you have ever been on an airplane ride and looked out the window, then you have probably noticed the ethereal world above the clouds.

It is so calm and relaxing, high off the ground, and far away from all of the stress of life.

Have you ever taken a ride in a hot air balloon?

Have you ever been lifted off the ground slowly, like you were being carried by a gentle giant to a restful place?

Your journey into peacefulness and relaxation will begin on the ground, preparing for your journey of slow and tender flight, as you crawl slowly through the clouds in a comfortable basket.

Begin your ascent first by laying down in a comfortable position.

If your body needs to be adjusted at all to help you for the most comfort in this space, make those adjustments now before you enter a place of total stillness.

You are going to be carried away on the air, firstly through your breath.

Your breath will align you with your inner harmony and balance.

Your breath will help fill you with the peacefulness you desire and help you release all of the cares and worries you may be carrying around with you right now.

Every inhale is a beautiful source [of comfort, refreshment, and light.

Every exhale is a letting go, a release of tension, a movement closer to restful relaxation.

Breathe here for a few moments.

Connect to your body.

Connect to your feelings.

Connect to the sense of relief from your breath…

You are here to feel free from the world of deadlines and agendas.

You are here to only exist within yourself and your deeper sense of true peace and balance.

This practice of connecting to your physical body through your breath, and your spiritual essence through your creative mind, is what will help you to refresh your life-force energy and feel fully healed, refreshed and connected to your inner soul.

Your only purpose now is just to float through a heavenly landscape.

Underneath your body, you begin to feel the softness of grass on a majestic hillside.

It is a bright and beautiful, sunny day.

As you look up into the sky, you can see that it is full of the most glorious, puffy, white clouds.

You are going to feel those clouds soon, gliding through and above them with the magic of your higher consciousness.

The soft grass around you is yielding, comforting, and pleasurable on your skin.

The warm sunlight feels just right, and the very subtle, gentle breeze is just right...for a hot air balloon ride...

You look over now and see the basket just walking distance away—the basket that will carry you far off into the heavens.

You are eager to go over to it and witness the gigantic balloon rise up off the ground, full of the hot air that will lift you up.

The basket is easy for you to climb into a much larger than you would have thought.

There is enough room inside for you to lay down in any direction.

The balloon is airing up while you are climbing inside.

It is starting to lift off of the grassy earth and align with the basket, to float over and hover above it.

You can feel yourself feeling elated but calm—excited, but relaxed.

Your path is up and up and up, and there is no other landscape, but the clouds on high.

You will get there soon.

Your balloon is almost ready to lift you up, and all you have to do when the time comes is pull on the cord to send you off the ground.

Inhale deeply, slowly pulling fresh air into your lungs...and exhale gently out.

Again, inhale slowly and steadily, gathering all of the hot air you will need to soar high up in the clouds...and exhale.

Breathe out all of the cares and worries that will weigh you down.

Breathe away all of the tension that will keep your balloon on the ground...

You are ready, and your balloon is ready.

It's time to pull the cord and feel your ascent.

The cord is easy to pull.

It feels effortless as you give it a tug and release hot air into the giant balloon above your head.

With one tug, you begin to feel your body in the basket, hover off the ground.

You pull the cord again and feel an even bigger lift off the grass.

You are now fully off the surface of the Earth with just a couple of tugs...

You can feel the pull upward.

It is smooth and slow.

Your hot air balloon can only go about 2 miles per hour.

There will be no speed on your journey.

You can take all the time you need to just feel pulled upward by the balloon and watch the world around you transform as you are carried higher and higher above the ground...

Your path is taking you further up.

The world below you becomes smaller as you ascend at a snail's pace.

You look off to the east, and you see a river flowing smoothly.

You think to yourself how big it seems when you are standing right beside it, and how small it seems now that you are floating high above it...

The river is full of life, and it flows smoothly, cutting across the land as far as the eye can see, the sunlight of the day glistening on its surface.

The river becomes smaller and smaller as you float higher and higher, taking a deep breath in and exhaling gently...

You look to the west, and you see a great, wide forest that pushes far across the land.

The trees seem infinite, endless.

As you glide high above the trees, you feel like you can hear the rustle of every squirrel, every bird, every forest creature rummaging for food.

There is no space between the horizon and the trees.

It stretches on forever...

The higher you go, the smaller the trees become, the wood of the branches and trunks disappearing behind the green foliage.

The tops of the trees, which once seemed so close, are now at a great distance from your hot air balloon.

You can feel the journey getting steadily closer to the clouds...

You look out of the basket to the south, and you see fields and meadows reaching far across the land, sewing a patchwork quilt of land as far as your eye can see to the south.

The lands of the farmers, the cattle, the goats and the sheep—the land of food that grows, of harvests and abundance from the fertile soil.

This land will stretch out for miles more, as your balloon gets ever higher, and can see that much farther across the land.

You look out to the north and are much higher now.

You begin to see the curve of the Earth from this height and feel completely restful as you look to the north star, already visible from this height in the sky.

You have ascended to the atmosphere of the cloud world, and it is here that you will find your greatest peacefulness and comfort.

It is here that you can let all of your worries and cares drift off and away from you, falling back to the earth as you drift through the clouds...

Look around you as you inhale deeply and exhale smoothly.

You are completely surrounded by puffs of white moisture.

They look like giant cotton balls piled together in beautiful mounds of softness.

You can no longer see the surface of the earth.

You are too high above the clouds now and can only see a great plain of white in every direction you face...

Your basket is moving slowly, but you feel the momentum of your balloon as it wafts on the breeze of the high atmosphere.

You have no trouble breathing here.

You can take deep, fulfilling breaths.

You can feel totally relaxed as you inhale and exhale from this point in the sky...

Breathe now as you let in the magnificent scenery of an all-white horizon fill your soul.

Breathe into this place of total calm and serenity.

Let the clouds high above the earth; comfort you.

You are warm here.

You are safe.

You have enough oxygen to breathe.

All you have to do is take in the majesty of this place.

The whole world above the clouds looks like a tundra of snow and ice for thousands of miles.

It looks angelic and full of bright light, the light from the sun reflecting off of the cloud faces.

Beneath the clouds is the whole landscape of the world you know—the world where you eat, sleep, work, love...

This place high above the earth, beyond the clouds, is where you can come to be to feel refreshed, relaxed, a sense of internal peace, and quiet.

You are not going to need any of your worries and fears up here.

All of your doubts, complaints about your daily life or work life, anything that is causing you stress, can be released from this hot air balloon ride...

Take a moment to consider this: what are you worried about today?

What has been causing you stress or discomfort?

Can you name it?

Can you make it specific?

What is the one thing that has been on your mind of late?

Let it come fully into your thoughts.

As you let it take shape in your thoughts, turn it into something you can hold in your hand, a physical object that represents this worry or stress…

It could be a heavy bag of sand that represents the weight that you feel from your work or your home life.

It could be a dollhouse to symbolize how you feel about your home or your living space.

It could be a person that has been upsetting you or weighing you down.

Anything is possible from this place within your mind.

Do not judge yourself for how it comes up or how it forms.

Simply allow it to take shape so that you can hold it in your hands…

Notice the clouds again and the atmosphere you are floating again.

Reminding yourself of your stress may have brought up those feelings for you again.

Look out to the clouds.

You are here in a hot air balloon, free to just release the pain you are suffering, free to align with your highest consciousness and internal vibration of light

Here you are, high above the clouds, facing your current anxiety or worry.

You are holding it in your hands, and you are ready to let it go.

You can hold it over the side of the balloon and prepare to let it go.

You are not hurting it, whatever it is.

It is a symbolic release of what has been holding you back from your relaxation and relief.

It is a symbolic action to cut the cords with your tension, worry, and doubt...

Hold the symbolic object over the edge and promise to let go of everything right here, right now.

You have no reason to hold onto this part of your life anymore.

You have no reason to doubt yourself.

You have no reason to fear to let go of this issue or these fears.

It is time.

Here, high above the clouds, it is time for you to say farewell to this part of your life.

It serves no purpose.

It only causes distress and discomfort.

Let it go.

Let it fall far away, through the clouds to wherever it must go.

Relieved to know that you are free of it.

Release it fully and take a nice, long breath in through your nose.

Hold your breath here for a moment, like you were holding the object over the side of the basket...and release the breath, letting it flow away from you.

Notice the serene landscape around you, unfolding as far as your eye can see...

You are safe here.

You are free.

You have released your discomfort.

You can now relax a little more and let yourself delve more deeply into your unconscious thoughts and dreams.

Here in the heavens, high above the soft, cotton-like clouds, you can prepare for your ascent farther and deeper into dreamland.

You will not return to the Earth tonight.

Tonight, you will continue to float high above the ground in your hot air balloon and find all of the relief you have been looking for.

Perhaps you have another object you want to release and toss over the side of the basket.

You can do that now.

You can take a moment to reflect on whatever happens to come up for healing.

Let it take shape and form in your mind.

Let it become something you can hold in your hands so that you can fully release it into the atmosphere, cutting ties with whatever has been weighing you down...

As you take a moment to do this, continue with your soothing breath, high up in the clouds.

Don't let go of the landscape that has been giving you so much comfort.

You are safe here.

You cannot fall.

You cannot be harmed.

You can breathe easily here.

You will find all of the relief you need simply by existing in this place high above the Earth.

The total calm and serenity of this world is what calms you and puts your heart at ease.

It is the place that prepares you for your dreams tonight.

It is the place that calls you home to your most comfortable and relaxed body, mind, and spirit.

You have everything you need now.

You are free to drift off, farther and farther into the clouds...farther and farther into your subconscious thoughts...farther and farther into the great beyond...the land of your dreams...

Float away...high on the clouds...float away... with your breath slow and steady...float away...with your heart full of peace...sweet dreams...

Chapter 10: Taking Flight in Dreamland

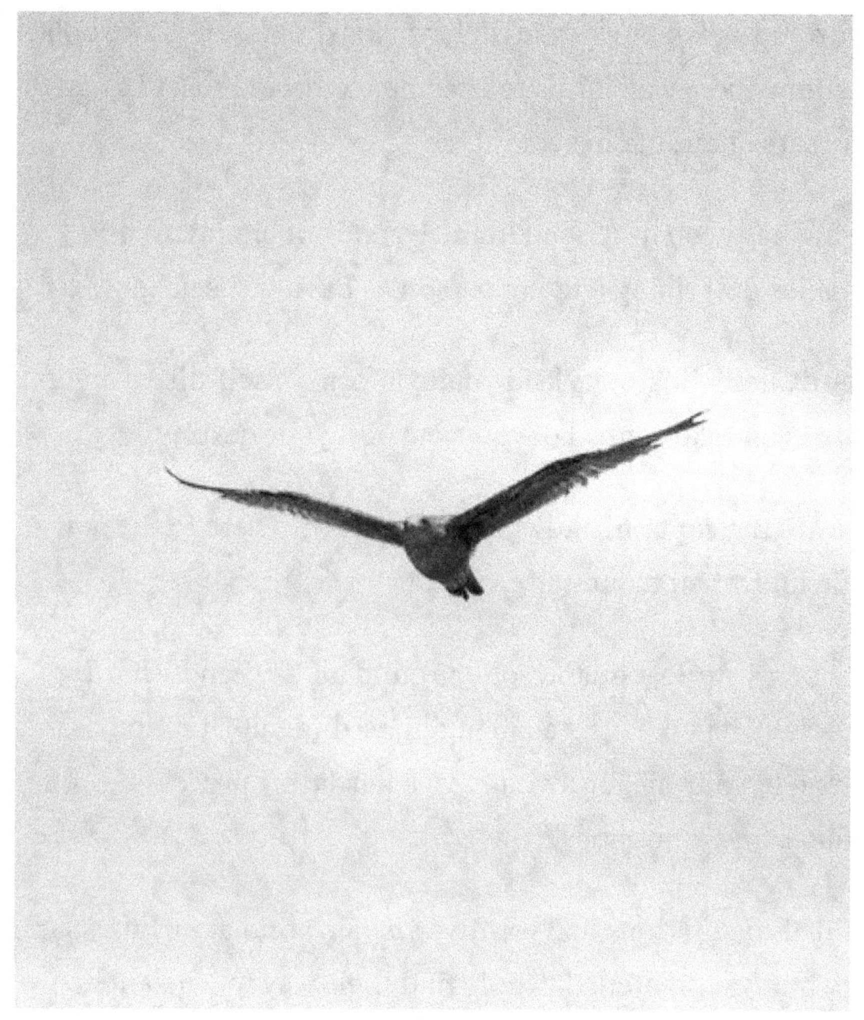

Almost all of us have had a dream that we are flying. Sometimes you have wings.

Sometimes you are just gliding through the air like a superhero.

Often times, when we take flight in our dreams, it is symbolic of freedom and a way for us to become connected to letting go of our fears about life in general.

Flying has been described in the legends of old myths and folktales describing a flying person as having special powers.

These tales will always lead you to a form of self-discovery in which you take control of your journey, your destiny.

You are the captain, and you know exactly where to fly, how high, and when to land.

Planting your feet on the solid ground all day can be hard, especially if you have a challenging or difficult situation or people in your life, or if you have a hard time processing your feelings and emotions.

Guided meditations and creative visualization are a huge part of how many enlightened people find their way to wholeness.

Your inner journey is just as valuable, meaningful, and important as your inner one.

When you follow your journey forward and trust yourself to fly in the right direction for yourself, then the stresses of life naturally fall away, and you can find peace, harmony, and balance with your whole life.

So take a moment to connect with this positive notion.

Find your comfort zone, and let yourself fall into freely.

You are here to enjoy your life journey, not stress out about it all of the time.

You are here to have a purpose that is meaningful to you, not worry about whether or not you are doing a good enough job, or if you are successful enough.

You have always been and always are enough, and when you acknowledge that truth...that's when you can really fly.

Find your most comfortable position.

Find the parts of your body that feel restless or tense and shake them out.

Shake out any part of your body that has felt motionless for far too long.

Shake off anything that you might have absorbed from another person today, or from a challenging experience.

Shake off all of the drama that finds you when you are trying to find your peace of mind...

Inhale deeply and enjoy the way it feels to have control over your breath.

Exhale slowly and appreciate the way it feels to let go of something physically from your body.

Inhale slowly again, rejoicing in the fresh air that fills you up.

Exhale slowly and feel gratitude that you have come to this place of self-healing, to totally bond with your own creative inspiration and thoughts, to become even more closely connected to your inner self, free of drama, free of critique...no judgments.

Your breath has helped your body feel more relaxed.

You are sinking more deeply into your comfort and relaxation.

You are finding it easier to breathe naturally and smoothly.

You are feeling content to just be present here, taking good care of yourself, giving yourself all of the love, attention, and devotion that you need right now...

There are no rules on your inner journey.

All you have to do is appreciate your creative ability to see more clearly from your inner world. Sometimes, all you need is to go within to find your answers and take flight, resolving all of your problems, issues, and challenges from your wise internal self...your higher self.

You are fully relaxed as you continue to breathe and let yourself take comfort in your personal power and light from within.

You may feel like you have already done this before, and that's okay.

You don't have to think about any of it—you just have to let yourself follow along, listen to the guided story, and enjoy the pleasure of flying...

You can see yourself clearly now.

You are looking at your reflection in a mirror or a window.

You can see your face, your features, your outfit.

How would you like to feel right now?

Do you feel the way you look in your reflection within your mind?

Do you look the way that you hope to feel?

As you gaze at your inner reflection, show yourself how you want to appear to yourself.

Give yourself the costume or uniform, the style or outfit that best suits how you want to feel within tonight.

You can change your hairstyle.

You can wear something you would normally never choose to put on in public.

Take a few moments as you breathe to appreciate the world you know in your mind.

You can be all of yourself here.

Allow yourself to appear the way you would like to feel right now...

You are going to feel like this for the rest of your guided meditation.

This is your world, and you can look and dress; however, you see fit.

You can change your outfit anytime you want to.

You can become whatever you really are deep down inside.

You might become an animal or a tree.

You might become a warrior or a princess.

You might become something that this world has never know before.

Enjoy the work of dressing yourself to fly.

When you are ready, inhale deeply...hold the breath for a count of three...and steadily release the breath from your body...

You are climbing up a staircase now.

It is made of stone, and it is carved as a spiral, going higher and higher.

It looks like the stairs within an ancient castle.

The castle is a part of your subconscious mind.

It is a place you can come to any time you need to in order to dress yourself the way you want to or hope to feel inside and out...

The stairs are taking you up to the top of the castle.

When you get to the rooftop, you are able to walk out onto it.

The castle overlooks a great and vast kingdom.

It is familiar to you.

You have traveled here before.

As you look out over the land, you can point out to yourself other places you have already been: in a meadow, in a forest, by the ocean on a ship, in the clouds, by a river, in a garden of wonders...

This place holds the secret truth of you and your inner journey.

The landscape is wholly yours, and you can be anything here and do anything you want to help yourself find your truth and purpose.

It is where you will return as you quest for deeper meaning in your life, as you seek to know who you really are, deep down inside...

Standing on the castle roof, taking in the inner world of your mind, you are now able to take a new journey.

From here in your kingdom, you can fly anywhere.

You are dressed to be how you want to feel, you have all of your inner power and life-force to guide you and you can fly over everything and everyone to get to your space of balance, harmony, and equality with the life you want to be living...

The flight will take you far, and the point of your journey now is to let your intuition guide you.

Your inner wisdom is what can help you find what you need to see right now, to help you relax and find peace of mind and inner calm.

You can let yourself find the right path when you trust yourself that you already know the answers.

You already know how to solve all of your problems, and you can find it all right here in this inner kingdom of your body, mind, heart, and soul...

To take flight, all you have to do is face the world you have created in your thoughts and mind.

Take a moment to breathe and relax into this visual journey.

Take a moment to connect with your breath again and let yourself feel that moment before you take flight...

Stepping closer to the roof's edge, imagine you are outstretching your arms like they are wings, stretching far out to either side of you.

Underneath you are just castle grounds...or is it a waterfall that leads through a great misty fog that goes to another place in your kingdom?

When you look down, you see not the grounds of a castle, but a portal into another place and you can fly there, just by leaping off the rooftop and finding your flight.

The waterfall drops off into another place you cannot see.

It is where you can begin to teach yourself how to journey within your mind.

You can imagine anything you want...anything at all.

You can see beyond the reality of Earth and look at your inner universe with creativity and imagination.

You can picture a rainbow bridge to fly over that will lead you to another part of your kingdom.

You can picture a flying Pegasus who will transport you wherever you want to go.

Here, in your kingdom, there are no rules.

You are the one who decides how your world will look and how you will find your way forward...

So, now, here in this place, prepare to take flight.

Your arms are spread.

Your outfit is just right.

You are relaxed, calm, and free to be anything you want...

Push off and fly...go wherever your intuition is guiding you.

You will not fall.

You will not be hurt.

You have the ability to fly in this place, and you are free to make your way through this world with your secret wing-span.

As you take flight and your world opens up to you more, what do you find?

What can you see?

Are there others here?

Are there new lands yet to be explored—more hidden caves and majestic gardens?

More cozy cottages deep in the woods, or ships to be sailed over your own, private ocean?

Are you joined by any animal guides?

Enjoy flying over your inner kingdom, and let keep unfolding for you.

Breathe steadily.

You can land anywhere you want and take off anywhere you want.

You are flying in order to get a bigger picture, greater scope, and nothing is too big or too small here. It is everything you ask it to be.

[give plenty of time for creative visualization and meditation here]

Your world is an awakening place.

It helps you find your creative life-force, your deeper truth, your secret purpose.

This world within your mind is a sacred landscape, a dimension of your thoughts and your feelings, to be explored like a great adventurer seeking hidden treasure in every cave, forest, and hideaway...

Bringing your focus back to your breath.

Let yourself continue exploring in ways you may not have before.

Let yourself delve more deeply into these ascended places.

Who do you meet along the way?

Have you met another spirit guide or ascended master who comes to teach you a lesson of healing and spiritual wisdom?

Do you have any specific places that you feel more draw to in this unique universe?

Wherever you are in your flight, give yourself a moment to see if you can find your castle again from this point of view.

Can you tell where you are on the map of your mind?

Are there secret tunnels and portals that will lead you right back to your castle?

Begin to find your way back to the castle now, breathing steadily and slowly along the way.

You can see it, and it feels far, but you have the ability to fly.

It won't take long to get there.

You are feeling more peaceful now and ready to fall fast asleep.

Your journey through the kingdom has shown you much and given you mush to appreciate.

You will find your sense of relaxation and restfulness more fully now.

You will feel ready to align with your dreaming mind and drift further and further into sleep...

The castle is drawing nearer, and you feel yourself preparing to land.

You have a strong body and are good at landing from your own flight.

It is like a dance, graceful and angelic.

The castle roof welcomes you back with ease, and you feel powerfully connected to your higher nature.

You follow your original path back to the mirror where you first began.

Down, down, down the stone steps of the castle, like you are unwinding...

As you come to the mirror again, you see your eyes again, your face, your body.

You see your outfit.

It may have changed, and that's okay.

Or perhaps, after flying through your inner world, you are ready to take on a new form.

How do you want to dress now, as you prepare for a wholesome night of gentle, peaceful rest?

What would feel best to you right now after feeling the freedom of flight?

Take a few moments and breaths to see yourself in the castle mirror...

Now, you are ready.

You can now retire in your inner kingdom, in the castle of your dreams and imagination.

Not far from your looking glass is a large bed, fit for a queen or king.

It has the softest sheets and blankets, the deepest most relaxing pillows, and it is all for you, waiting for you, warm and inviting.

You walk over and climb your way up to the large mattress, tucking your legs under the covers, feeling silk against your skin.

You can finally rest after a long flight and journey around your kingdom.

As you snuggle in, long, heavy velvet curtains are pulled closed around the bed, wrapping you in comfort and deep, luxurious peacefulness.

You are free to disappear into your dreams now.

Your work is done.

You are here to rest all the way, deep into the world of the unconscious...

Release your breath...feel held by the magic of your castle, your kingdom, your inner world...you can fly anywhere you want, even all the way into your dreams.

You are floating into your dreams now, soft and serene, high up in your castle, safe, wrapped in velvet and silk...

Dream that you are flying over your kingdom again...peacefully, serenely, calmly...sweet dreams.

Conclusion

Thank you for making time for *Bedtime Stories for Adults* and let's hope it was helpful and able to provide you with all of the tools you need to achieve your goals whatever they may be.

Your journey of centeredness, wholeness, and balance will move forward as you continue to support yourself through these meditation practices.

You can use them anytime you need to in order to find the restfulness you are looking for.

Or to help you unravel and unwind your thoughts and begin to rejoice in the feeling of total relaxation.

The best part of using these tools and resources is that you are able to change your present state of anxiety, tension, worry, or stress in a matter of minutes.

Just by shutting off the outside world for a few minutes, going within and exploring your deeper mind and consciousness.

Acquiring the self-healing tools, you need to feel refreshed every day and every night.

You can begin to achieve the calmness of mind, body, and spirit that lifts you higher and higher into your truest state of being.

Allowing you to fully rest and replenish your energy, helping you to feel prepared for anything life hands you.

Continue to work with these guided meditations as a way to find comfort, peace of mind, and healing power from within.

Bedtime Stories for Adults will give you all of the serenity and soothing comfort you need to fall asleep, heal your mind and spirit, and find your wholeness every day.

Finally, if you found these meditations useful in any way, a review on Amazon is always appreciated!

<u>You might also be interested in</u>

Bedtime Stories for Stressed-Out Adults: Fantasy stories and poems for stress relief and a good night of relaxed sleep. Lullabies for grown-ups.

www.ingramcontent.com/pod-product-compliance
Lightning Source LLC
Chambersburg PA
CBHW070659250726

48662CB00001B/198